THE VEGAN ATHLETE

THE VEGAN ATHLETE

BEN GREENE and BRETT STEWART

Maximizing Your Health & Fitness While
Maintaining a Compassionate Lifestyle

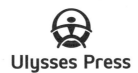

Ulysses Press

Published in the United States by
Ulysses Press
P.O. Box 3440
Berkeley, CA 94703
www.ulyssespress.com

ISBN13: 978-1-61243-132-1
Library of Congress Control Number 2012951896

Printed in the United States by Bang Printing

10 9 8 7 6 5 4 3 2 1

Acquisitions Editor: Keith Riegert
Managing Editor: Claire Chun
Editor: Lily Chou
Proofreader: Lauren Harrison
Index: Sayre Van Young
Design and layout: what!design @ whatweb.com
Interior photographs: © Rapt Productions except pages 65 and 75 © Brett Stewart
Cover photographs: quinoa © Foodpictures/shutterstock.com; man © Kzenon/shutterstock.com; woman
    © Aleksandr Markin/shutterstock.com; edamame © ponsulak kunsub/shutterstock.com; butternut squash
    © sarsmis/shutterstock.com
Models: Lewis Elliot, Evan Klontz, Brett Stewart

Please Note

This book has been written and published strictly for informational and educational purposes only, and in no way should be used as a substitute for consultation with health care professionals. You should not consider educational material herein to be the practice of medicine or to replace consultation with a physician or other medical practitioner. You should always consult with your physician before altering or changing any aspect of your medical treatment and/or undertaking a diet regimen, including the guidelines as described in this book. The author and publisher are providing you with information in this work so that you can have the knowledge and can choose, at your own risk, to act on that knowledge. The author and publisher also urge all readers to be aware of their health status and to consult health care professionals before beginning any health or diet program.

This book is dedicated to my family—Mom, Dad, Bryan, Jonathan, Dominic, Sidney and Bailey.
I love you guys more than I could ever express with words!
—Ben

Dear Mom, you were right about the broccoli.
—Brett

TABLE OF CONTENTS

FOREWORD

Hi, I'm Brett from 7weekstofitness.com, and I've been lucky enough to publish quite a few fitness books with some amazing professional athletes, trainers, nutritionists and coaches. Being a fitness author, I'm surrounded by healthy and passionate individuals of all ages who represent all levels of fitness, and each one has a story to tell and a lesson to teach. At 42 years old, I can confidently say I'm the fittest I've ever been thanks to tips, tricks and sound fitness and nutritional advice I've learned from my coauthors, training partners, friends and clients. While I've never officially been a practicing veg*n (vegetarian or vegan), when I met my coauthor Ben Greene for the first time, I knew my life would change forever. Ben is a bright, young, energetic athlete whose love for the sport of triathlon and passion for being a vegan was introduced to me by a mutual friend; along with that chance encounter came a wealth of knowledge about eating more healthily, treating my body—and not coincidentally the Earth—with more respect and developing a deeper connection with the choices I make when I'm fueling my body for training, racing or even daily activities. Ben practices what he (quietly) preaches, and has the physique and success as a trainer and athlete to back it up.

The addition of Corey Irwin, a running coach, athlete and outstanding chef with an unstoppable drive for tinkering with and perfecting recipes to the max, was extremely fortuitous as she was just beginning to write her own series of cookbooks. We were lucky enough to get some of her time (OK, hundreds of hours) to devote to the delicious vegan recipes you'll find throughout the book. Corey's popularity online and in print as a contributor to many publications was an added bonus, as her devoted readers could share this journey along with Ben and me as we crafted this book.

Brett Stewart
Phoenix, Arizona
2013

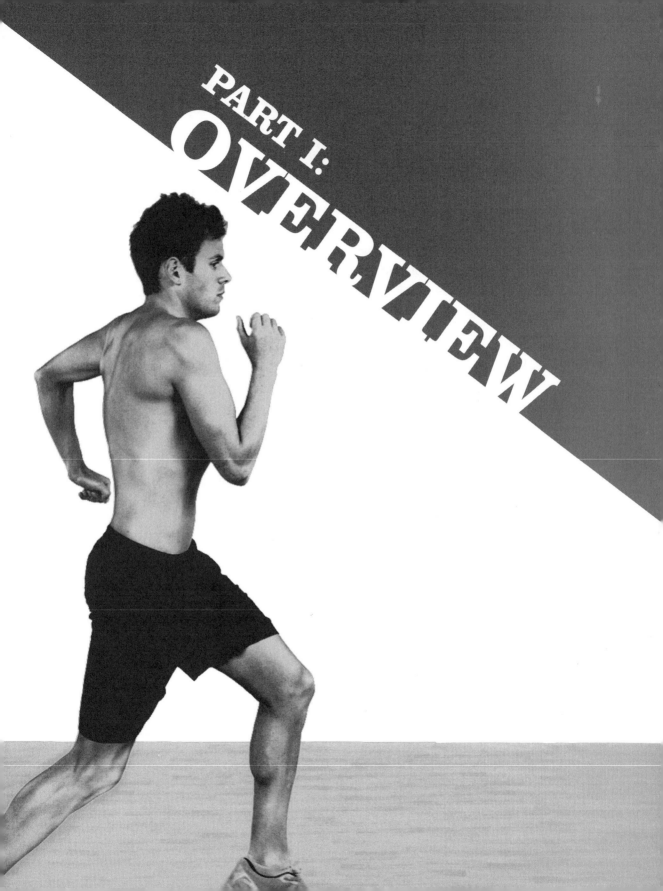

PART I: OVERVIEW

INTRODUCTION

"You are what you eat." Apparently, Mom knew what she was talking about—if only we would listen!

We've all heard that phrase and dismiss it as simple rhetoric. Even with tons of documentation from research and nutritional information right at our fingertips, most people fail to comprehend that simple statement and make the necessary correlation: The food we consume is such an important factor in our health, energy, well-being and ability to function on a daily basis that it should be chosen carefully based on intelligent, well-informed information.

There's no question that individuals living in the twenty-first century have in-depth data readily available about the nutritional values of certain foods and dangers of others. The disconnect lies in how few people actually spend the time to do even cursory research before deciding what to ingest. Every minute of every day, millions of people are turning a blind eye to the dangers of the foods they consume, whether it be by eating inherently unhealthy items that they "know" are bad for them or by unwittingly ingesting unseen pesticides, bacteria or hormones that lurk in their food choices.

From drive-thrus to fad diets, the overwhelming majority of individuals in modernized countries focus on the ease and convenience of food rather than the actual content of their meals. There are now generations of humans who have existed with convenience food in millions of different combinations. This societal shift has all but erased the decision-making process based on food availability or quality and replaced it with choices based on flavor: Do you want Thai or Mexican food?

The numbers behind the trends are staggering. On average, a single American consumes 200 pounds of meat, poultry and fish per year. Comparing that amount of ingested animal protein to what it was just 50 years ago, the increase is nearly 25 percent—or 50 pounds more per individual. Protein intake has ballooned to approximately 110 grams per day (nearly double what the USDA recommends for healthy, active adults), with nearly 80 percent of those amino acids coming from animal flesh, eggs and dairy.

Not coincidentally, the average weight of Americans has risen steadily over the last five decades by approximately 25 pounds, and obesity has run rampant throughout our society. Males of nearly 200 pounds and females of 165 pounds (just 35 pounds less) have become the norm, with many nutritionists attributing this weight gain to our penchant for eating animal proteins three times per day, at an average of a half-pound total.

While statistics and definitions vary widely from nation to nation, less than 16 percent of the 7 billion people on this planet consider themselves vegetarian—subsisting entirely on a plant-based diet without ingesting any animal protein. The Asian subcontinent contributes extensively to that percentage, with some areas of India adhering to a nearly 100-percent vegetarian diet. Vegans make up a small but growing portion of the vegetarians around the world; by some accounts, the number is higher than 1 percent of Earth's population. While 1 percent may not seem like an incredibly significant number, it's enough to make up an entire army—literally. In the United States, with a population of 313 million, the 3.1 million vegans are nearly person for person the same number of individuals as all of the active-duty U.S. soldiers and their families. Vegans and vegetarians (or veg*ns, the combined moniker that's gaining a great deal of popularity through online and social channels) are a significant, influential group whose numbers are continuing to rise. Their message is also gaining immense popularity across the globe: Humans do not need to eat animal flesh to survive, thrive or even become superstar athletes.

In *The Vegan Athlete*, we'll share the journey of a certified personal trainer and Ironman triathlete's journey into becoming vegan while competing at the highest levels of physical endurance, strength and speed. We'll also share two dozen delicious vegan recipes, created by an award-winning chef, that are extremely nutritious and deliver the protein needed for an active, athletic individual to get lean and strong while following the goals-based training and fitness programs created specifically for this book.

ABOUT THIS BOOK

Reading this book won't turn you into a vegan. It may change your perspective, give you some clarity on the hows and whys of the vegan lifestyle and open your eyes to some extremely valuable nutritional lessons, but when you close the cover and put this book on your coffee table, you won't be transformed into a vegan, veg*n, vegetarian or similar. This book is neither a preachy tome dedicated to turning the human population into vegans nor the rantings of a few athletes screaming from a soapbox about how meat-eaters are turning the world into a hell and destroying our planet. Rather, this is an informational book replete with stories, tips, tricks, a boatload of recipes, three goal-specific fitness programs, and a nutritional regimen.

Part I of *The Vegan Athlete* begins with an overview featuring some statistics around common nutritional choices and the veg*n population worldwide, as well as some background on the authors and contributors of this book. The real-world transition of Ben Greene from a self-professed "meat-head" to a vegan endurance athlete showcases some of the ups and downs of making this lifestyle, nutrition and training switch, and is followed by a comprehensive explanation of the benefits of a vegan lifestyle, understanding the perceived social stigmas, success stories of some impressive athletes, and an introduction to fueling for athletic performance with food selections that anyone can easily follow. The FAQ section helps to dispel some of the misconceptions about the vegan lifestyle and also addresses proper everyday nutrition, fueling for sports performance and meal preparation and timing. We'll even share some tips on shopping for vegan foods.

Part II covers the health and athletic performance benefits of following a vegan diet and also addresses topics such as dealing with the arguments you may encounter when you become vegan, dietary considerations and foods vegans should be aware of. You'll find nutritional advice on fueling for high performance in training and events, during travel, and even recovery after the big race. An easy-to-follow "Beginner's 3-Step Guide to Going Vegan" for those interested in trying a vegan diet is followed by a "2 Weeks to Eat Like a Vegan" meal plan with tons of unique meals, drinks and snacks to choose from.

Part III contains three different training programs, each with a different goal (weight loss, strength, endurance), with two corresponding workout routines for each goal based on your existing level of fitness.

Each four-week program also features nutrition tips tailored to each training regimen to help you reach your health, fitness and athletic performance goals.

In the Appendix you'll find 20 tantalizing recipes created by chef, athlete and running coach Corey Irwin, all reviewed and tested by certified personal trainer, triathlete and vegan athlete Ben Greene. Along with the step-by-step recipes, you'll also find a helpful chart to make veganizing your favorite recipes a snap by replacing traditional ingredients with vegan-friendly alternatives.

BEN'S VEGAN JOURNEY

Growing up, I ate meat fairly regularly. Like most Americans (and being a kid), I didn't have much choice in what I ate. If my parents cooked it, I ate it—at least most of the time. As I grew older, I became more interested in overall health. I also began to lift weights and I was soon determined to develop as much muscle as I possibly could. My nutritional regimen (if you could call it that) consisted of eating everything in my sight—entire jars of peanut butter, dozens of cheeseburgers—and I eventually developed my 5'8" frame up to 160 pounds.

After I graduated high school and grew out of my self-proclaimed "meat-head" phase, I found endurance athletics. Proper nutrition is key in endurance sports, so I started to play around with my own diet to see what worked best for me. I grew up on a small farm and have always loved animals. Over time my compassion for animals began to win me over; it became harder and harder for me to eat meat for personal reasons, and I became a vegetarian in 2008.

My older brother Dominic played a big part in my dietary change, as he had transformed from a meat eater to a vegan only a few years earlier and had nothing but positive things to say about his lifestyle change. I was amazed at how quick and seemingly effortless the transition was for him and decided that becoming a vegetarian was the right choice for me.

Going v*gan is not a choice that someone can make for you; it's a choice that I believe should come naturally and is something that you need to decide for yourself. As I started to do more research on how animal products affect the human body, I began to realize that animal products aren't optimal for how I want to fuel my body or live my life.

In early 2009, I decided to become a strict vegan and put a great deal of time and effort into making choices that supported my new goals. However, I failed miserably. I was unsuccessful in completing the transition basically because I didn't have the dedication and passion for living a vegan lifestyle. While going vegan is very simple to do and, when done correctly, can work wonders on your overall health, it's not just a switch that can be flipped and will take a differing amount of time for each individual. For my brother it was relatively quick, while for me it took nearly a year of renewed effort.

After about three years of being a strict vegetarian, I became a dedicated vegan athlete in 2010. An online video called "Meet Your Meat" was the impetus. After seeing how poorly animals are treated during the entire process, I vowed to never eat another animal product again. A big reason I went vegan was because I wanted my diet to reflect my nonviolent beliefs. As someone who always preaches nonviolence, I was ashamed to realize how much violence there was in my old diet. Once I dedicated myself to going vegan, during my second attempt I found it relatively easy for me to successfully make the transition. As a vegetarian I'd already cut out most animal products, so the changes didn't shock me too much. For many individuals, the concept of becoming vegan seems hard or scary, but the reality of the transformation is usually far less difficult than they expect. We're all such incredibly different individuals and each vegetarian or vegan lifestyle adaptation will take its own course and period of time.

Since going 100 percent vegan, my body and mind have never felt better. Training for and competing in events like the Ironman-distance triathlons requires a lot of time, patience and discipline, but it also taxes your body a great deal too. Being vegan has been very beneficial for my training and development as an endurance athlete; I'm able to recover more quickly, train longer and maintain my focus for prolonged periods of time. I attribute my refined mental and physical focus to my vegan lifestyle and healthy vegan diet.

FAQS ANSWERED BY BEN GREENE

Q. *What do vegans eat?*

A. Being vegan means that you don't consume any animal products at all. It's easier to answer this question with a list of things that vegans don't eat: meat, fish, fowl, eggs, dairy, gelatin and other animal products. Many people believe that vegan food is bland and boring, but that simply isn't true. Maintaining a vegan diet opens up each individual's ability to become more creative with food and spices. Check out the recipes starting on page 90 for plenty of culinary creativity and insight into cooking vegan.

Q. *Is a vegan diet more expensive than a non-vegan diet?*

A. Yes and no. Maintaining a vegan diet can be very cheap if you buy certain foods in bulk, but your grocery bill can become very expensive when purchasing prepackaged foods and organically grown produce. Quite often "organic" or "vegan" on a label begets a significantly higher price tag. Fresh produce is your best bet to keep healthy food on your plate and some green in your wallet.

Q. *Where do vegans get their protein?*

A. This is the question that most if not all vegetarians and vegans are sick of hearing. In most developed countries, getting enough protein is not an issue. Many plants contain high amounts of protein. Some great plant-based proteins include beans, nuts, grains, seeds, tofu, nut milks … the list could go on. If you maintain a healthy and balanced plant-based diet, you'll have no problem getting enough protein.

While protein deficiency is very rare in America, some common symptoms include brittle or thinning hair, edema, hyperpigmentation of the skin, muscle weakness, muscle decay, a protruding belly and skin rashes. Eating too little protein compromises your normal immune activity, leaving you more susceptible to illness. Chronic protein deficiency may cause comas, shock or permanent physical disability.

Q. Isn't being vegan a little extreme? Why not just be vegetarian?

A. There are many reasons why people become vegan. Most people either have moral, health or environmental reasons for doing so. Some moral reasons could include the terrible treatment of animals that are kept for slaughter. Another reason people choose veganism over vegetarianism is for the health benefits of maintaining a plant-based diet. This will be explained throughout the book. The final reason would be for the environment, in that the production of animal products for human consumption causes a big amount of pollution.

"A recent United Nations report concluded that a global shift toward a vegan diet is necessary to combat the worst effects of climate change. And the U.N. is not alone in its analysis. Researchers at the University of Chicago concluded that switching from a standard American diet to a vegan diet is more effective in the fight against climate change than switching from a standard American car to a hybrid." ~PETA.org

Q. Is being vegan hard?

A. Being vegan is not hard at all. Cooking vegan food is just as easy as cooking non-vegan food; in fact, it might even be a lot easier. However, changing a habit is always hard; it takes time to make the change. One big piece of advice to someone who's afraid to go vegan because of all of the foods that you'll no longer be able to eat is to take it slowly. For your first week you can eliminate milk. Then the next week eliminate eggs and so forth. Some people easily go vegan when they learn about the exploitation of animals for food. Knowing about this suffering and exploitation made it impossible for Ben not to become vegan.

Q. Is it harder to cook vegan food?

A. Creating and cooking any meal can be as difficult or as hard as you make it. Being vegan just means you choose your ingredients more carefully. Most vegan cooking is actually a lot easier. When you cook with animal products, you need to be very careful to make sure that the food is cooked properly to kill all of the bacteria. If animal products aren't cooked properly, salmonella can be transmitted to the consumer of the food. Salmonella is present on raw meat and poultry, and can survive if the product isn't cooked to a safe minimum internal temperature (as measured with a food thermometer). When cooking vegan, you'll still need to make sure to wash all fruits and vegetables thoroughly before eating them, but you'll remove all the fears of meat-borne bacteria or parasites.

Q. Does it take longer to cook vegan food?

A. Generally speaking, cooking is cooking and creating a vegan meal takes no longer to make than a non-vegan selection. Of course, how complicated you choose to make the meal is completely up to you; using the recipes in this book will hopefully make you more creative and educated about ways to create dazzling meals for yourself, your family and your friends.

Q. Humans are meant to eat meat. How can I survive without it?

A. Individuals can survive and thrive without eating meat; this is proven daily by millions of vegans and vegetarians worldwide. Some of the finest endurance athletes in the world train, compete and thrive on an entirely meat-free diet. From muscle-bound Hollywood actors to Olympic decathletes, the health and well-being of individuals who made the choice to subsist on a meat-free diet is a constant reminder that humans do not need to consume animal flesh to survive.

Of course, humans can eat meat. We're omnivores and can eat just about any plant and animal product as long as it's prepared properly (picked, plucked, cooked, shelled, shucked or slaughtered) but we're not specifically predestined to eat copious amounts of animal flesh. That's left up to true carnivores.

Q. What's a carnivore?

A. A carnivore is described as any animal that feeds on the flesh of other animals. While humans can and do eat animal flesh, we're omnivores, not true carnivores. The following are some critical distinctions between both:

Carnivores: Have claws to help rip apart other animals for consumption.

Humans: Do not have claws adapted for hunting. Humans had to create tools to kill animals. Before the invention of tools, it was too dangerous to hunt and kill animals so humans lived off the land by subsisting on wild fruits, berries, nuts, roots and anything our ancestors could find. The term "hunter-gatherer" is often used to describe early human nutrition, although it's probably more realistic to say our early ancestral roots came more from gathering, and then eventually hunting. Devoid of weapons or tools, the majority of human nutrition would still be predominantly described as "gathering." For direct evidence of this, watch any reality-based survival program and you'll find that "modern" man will search for sustenance off the land as the primary source of food for survival.

Carnivores: Have sharp front teeth for tearing, with no flat molar teeth for grinding.

Humans: Do not have sharp front teeth but do have flat molars for grinding up plant material prior to digestion. This is a trait shared with purely plant-eating animals, or herbivores.

Carnivores: Have strong hydrochloric acid in their stomach to digest meat. This means that the meat that they eat doesn't sit in their bodies for long. It's broken down and excreted much more quickly than it is in humans.

Humans: Have stomach acid that's 20 times weaker than that of a meat eater. This means that the meat that you ate yesterday or even five days ago may still be processing through your digestive tract. Comparatively, it takes the human body about six to eight hours to digest most fruits and vegetables.

Carnivores: Have an intestinal tract that's only three times their body length so that rapidly decaying meat can pass through quickly. This means that cholesterol, fat and other negative elements are not absorbed into the body.

Humans: Have an intestinal tract nearly ten to twelve times their torso length. During that roughly 30-foot journey, our intestines absorb nutrients from the foods that we eat. Since our intestines are longer, there's far more time and surface area to absorb all the bad things in meat that a true carnivore doesn't take in. Meat contains cholesterol and fat, which are very bad for humans and can cause high blood pressure, heart disease, high cholesterol and a slew of other problems for us.

Q. Will I lose weight by following a vegan diet?

A. Not necessarily. You can follow a vegan diet and still gain weight if you rely on a lot of processed prepackaged foods. When transitioning into a vegan lifestyle, meat replacement products are a great way to ease the transition from being a meat eater. However, these products aren't the healthiest option for you. To maintain a healthy body on a vegan diet, you need to keep a balanced diet that includes lots of fruits, vegetables and whole grains. A recent scientific review found that "a vegetarian diet is highly effective for weight loss. Vegetarian populations tend to be slimmer than meat eaters, and they experience lower rates of heart disease, diabetes, high blood pressure and other life-threatening conditions linked to overweight and obesity."

Q. Will maintaining a vegan diet improve the condition of my skin?

A. Yes, it will. Many vegetables and fruits contain carotenoids, which are compounds that are metabolized by our bodies into vitamin A. Vitamin A produces sebum, an oil that's key to healthy skin growth and vital for skin health. Carotenoids are plant pigments responsible for the red, orange and yellow colors of fruits and vegetables. Some sources of carotenoids or vitamin A include sweet potatoes, carrots, kale and spinach.

The standard American diet contains plenty of meat and dairy, which lead to acidification of the blood. This causes damage to the endothelial cells that line blood vessels. When endothelial cells are damaged, they lose some of their ability to expand and become less pliable. The blood vessels to our skin are lined with endothelial cells; when these are damaged, blood flow to our skin is reduced. This can lead to early signs of aging, like wrinkles. Every time you eat an animal product, you're putting a little more acid in your body, which wears down your body as a whole.

Q. What's the difference between a vegan and a vegetarian?

A. Many people often get these two different diets confused on a regular basis. Being a vegetarian can mean a lot of things, whether it's a lacto-ovo vegetarian, a pescatarian, a pollo vegetarian, an ovo vegetarian or a lacto vegetarian.

Total vegetarians eat only plant food; they don't eat any animal foods, including fish, eggs, dairy products and honey. Lacto-ovo vegetarians don't eat poultry, beef, fish, shellfish or animal flesh of any kind, but they do consume food that contains eggs and dairy. Since the exclusion of dairy and/or eggs can be extremely difficult for many people, this is probably the most popular form of vegetarianism; it's the least restrictive and the easiest to follow. Lacto-ovo vegetarians can also be split up into lacto vegetarians (those who consume dairy products) and ovo vegetarians (those who consume eggs).

Vegetarians who abstain from eating all meat and animal flesh with the exception of fish are called pescatarians. Individuals who adopt this kind of diet are on the rise as it's a healthier eating choice than being an omnivore and also can work as a stepping stone to a fully vegetarian or even vegan diet. Pollo vegetarians eat poultry, such as chicken, turkey and duck.

A fully vegan diet is the most restrictive of the vegetarian diets and means that you don't consume any animal products whatsoever—this means no eggs, dairy, fish or animal flesh of any kind. Adhering to a completely vegan diet requires abstaining from consuming anything that has been derived from an animal product, including trace elements of ingredients that are extremely common in many mainstream foods (page 43 features a list of some common ingredients and foods that vegans should beware of). A balanced vegan diet consists of consuming plenty of fresh fruits, vegetables, grains and legumes. Those who maintain this type of nutritional intake purport to reap numerous health benefits.

Vegans not only omit all animal products from their diets but also eliminate them from the rest of their lives. Vegans use nothing from animals, be it leather, wool or silk.

Ben: *"Being vegan surely doesn't mean your plate is bland; one thing that stood out to me most when I became vegan was the amount of color that I had on every plate of food that I ate."*

PART II:
BEING A VEGAN ATHLETE

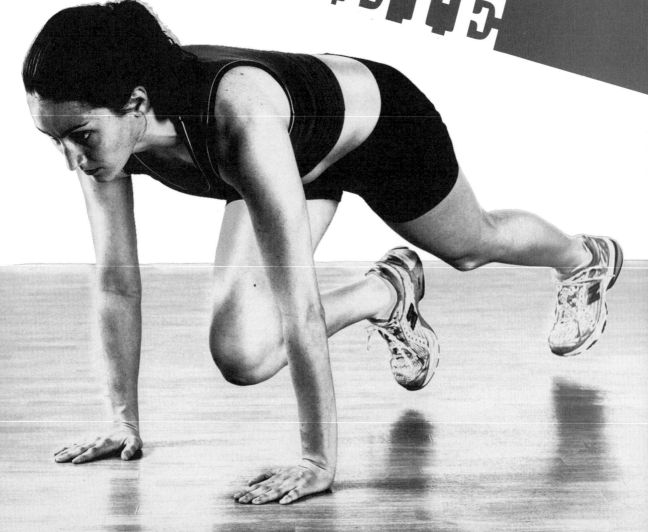

THE BENEFITS

We started this book with the familiar phrase "you are what you eat" for good reason—it has been used for over 250 years regarding the notion that to be fit and healthy you need to ingest healthy food. The first literal usage of this phrase came about in 1923, when nutritionist Victor Lindlahr was quoted (ironically in an ad for beef): "Ninety percent of the diseases known to man are caused by cheap foodstuffs. You are what you eat."

Nearly a century later we're still plagued with diseases that can be attributed to "cheap foodstuffs" but also the chemicals, preservatives, antibiotics, pesticides and even parasites that are present in the animal flesh that humans consume in large quantities year after year. In order to reduce the vast amount of artificial and harmful ingredients from their diet, over 60 million people worldwide choose to be vegetarian; approximately 1 million of those non meat eaters are vegans. In recent studies and surveys, the predominant reason why veg*ans choose their lifestyle and diet is to "improve their overall health by choosing a natural approach to wellness."

By removing the toxins associated with meat consumption, studies have shown that vegetarian and vegan diets can reduce the risks of cancer-based fatalities by as much as 50 percent while also ingesting the healthy foods that can slow or even halt the progression of the disease. According to the Physicians Committee for Responsible Medicine, vegetarians "are about 40 percent less likely to get cancer than non-vegetarians, regardless of other risks such as smoking, body size and socioeconomic status."

Oxidative stress on the body is yet another serious health issue that affects some consumers of animal products like dairy and meat. One of the major deleterious effects that meat eating has on our body is that it causes our bodies' pH levels to become overly acidic, which creates an environment in which bacteria and viruses can flourish, fatigue and malaise can overtake a normally healthy individual, and even cellular damage can begin to occur.

Every single food that we consume contains a natural substance called purines, which are essential for cellular health. Certain animal products (for example, chicken, beef, pork, most seafood) have a very high amount of purines. When a large amount of purines is consumed, our bodies metabolize this substance as uric acid. Uric acid is naturally found in our bodies and is necessary for a healthy body. Uric acid in our blood, for example, serves as an antioxidant and helps prevent damage to our blood vessel linings. Thus, a continuous supply of uric acid is important for protecting our blood vessels.

Improved Health

Many studies worldwide have shown that a veg*n diet is healthier and has a much lower risk of the following:

Prostate, ovarian, breast and colon cancer: An 11-year German study concluded as high as a 50 percent reduction in the risk of developing cancer by following a vegetarian diet.

Heart disease, high blood pressure, type 2 diabetes and stroke: These are all potentially reduced by removing red meat from the typical human diet. Studies have shown that as little as 3 ounces of unprocessed red meat daily can increase mortality rates up to 13 percent; with processed meat (hot dogs, etc.) that number balloons to 20 percent due to the concentration of nitrates and preservatives found in those products.

Osteoporosis: Cornell researchers found that individuals eating a plant-based diet helped to reduce the risk of osteoporosis versus those who consumed a diet high in animal protein, including dairy products. Even with the elevated levels of calcium found in dairy products, the high levels of animal protein actually leached more calcium from the bones than was ingested.

Many more health issues that we're not even aware of yet: Growth hormones, pesticides, antibiotics, preservatives and other unhealthy "ingredients" that are purposefully added to animal products all may have additional side effects that we're not aware of yet. Couple that with outbreaks of diseases that fester in animal slaughterhouses (such as mad cow disease), there's the extreme potential of very serious, adverse, long-term health effects by partaking in a heavily meat-based diet.

However, when we accumulate too much uric acid in our systems, we can develop problems like gout and kidney issues. Our kidneys are responsible for keeping our blood's uric acid levels balanced, but a meat-heavy diet can quickly overload them. When uric acid accumulates in our bodies, it crystallizes into what are called monosodium urate crystals. When these crystals accumulate they can become deposited in organs such as the kidneys as well as cause painful inflammation in joints, resulting in a condition referred to as gout.

A plant-based diet is extremely beneficial for endurance athletes (or everyone else, for that matter) in that plants are easily digested by our bodies and able to provide energy and nutrients quickly into the bloodstream. Quality sources of carbs, proteins and fats, plants are the perfect source for fuel for athletes who must maintain a healthy, lean-muscle-to-weight ratio in order to perform at their maximal potential. The less GI-intensive processing involved in plant-based intake results in optimum pre- and post-workout digestion, when an athlete's body needs the proper nutrition to fuel or repair muscles without diverting excessive blood flow to the stomach to laboriously process animal flesh.

Another major benefit of a plant-based diet for athletes is that it's highly conducive to healthy weight loss as well as the maintenance of a lower body weight, according to a 2006 study conducted by the Physicians Committee for Responsible Medicine. Vegetarian populations tend to be slimmer than meat eaters. They also experience lower rates of heart disease, diabetes, high blood pressure and other life-threatening conditions linked to overweight and obesity.

Endurance athletes always want to go faster and longer, and one effective way to do that is to lose some body fat. It's very simple: The lighter you are, the faster you'll be. To prove this point, just look at Isaac Newton's second law of motion, which states that acceleration is directly proportional to force and inversely proportional to mass. To illustrate this, here's an example: There are two runners, A and B, who are both 5'10" tall. Runner A is 150 pounds with a body fat of 12 percent, while runner B is 180 pounds with a body fat of 25 percent. Both runners' muscles can produce the same amount of force. Runner A will automatically be faster because the force generated by his muscles will be able to move his body more easily and with less effort, therefore making him faster and more efficient overall. Runner B will be slower because the amount of force generated has to move more mass overall.

Vegans' Reduced Impact on the Environment

Being vegan can be more than just what you eat. Many vegans also forgo wearing products that are made from animal products. Most of the clothes that you're wearing right now probably have some form of animal product in them, even if you're not wearing leather or fur. Many dyes, adhesives and materials are derived from animals. This is just another area to think about when you become vegan. Being vegan and eco-conscious generally go hand and hand. The production of meat and clothing causes a great amount of pollution that isn't needed in an already polluted world.

A 2012 article in *Leather International* states that "the tanning industry has been ranked as the fifth-worse polluting industry by the New York–based NGO Blacksmith Institute and the Green Cross." Leather is just one common fabric that Americans and the rest of the world consume on a mass level. The production of these goods not only harms the animals but they harm the people who work and live around the factories. Many goods that are produced and purchased in the U.S. are imported from around the world, many from third-world countries that don't have strict environmental controls like we do in the U.S. The lack of strict environmental controls leads to the improper disposal of waste products and other materials. The disposal of these waste products hurts the environment as well as the people who live near the factories and beyond. Before you take home that new leather jacket, it needs to be put through the tanning process. Tanning is the process of treating animal skins to produce leather. Once leather is tanned, it's more durable and less susceptible to decomposition. Chromium sulfate is a common chemical used in the commercial tanning industry. According to a report titled "The World's Worst Toxic Pollution Problems," chromium puts an estimated 1.8 million people worldwide at pollution risk.

Global warming has become a major issue over the past few years. Everyone from our government to our grandparents are talking about it. With the world's population growing larger on a daily basis, we'll need to produce more food. More than 70 percent of the grains that we grow in the U.S. are fed to animals that will be slaughtered for meat. It takes a whopping 16 pounds of grain to produce a single pound of meat! This doesn't seem like a very efficient system. If we were starving, we'd take the 16 pounds of grain any day over the 1 pound of meat. According to a 2001 U.S. Department of Agriculture report, "At present, the U.S. livestock population consumes more than 7 times as much grain as is consumed directly by the entire American population."

If nothing changes, the rate of starving and malnourished people in the world will balloon out of control. The United Nations Food and Agriculture Organization (FAO) estimates that "925 million people in the world are considered hungry all the time." That's 13.6 percent of the estimated world population of 6.8 billion. Note that "hungry" doesn't mean that they simply want a snack! "Hungry" is defined as "the uneasy or painful sensation caused by want of food; craving appetite. Also the exhausted condition caused by want of food." Most of you reading this book probably have never experienced true hunger before. The current system that we're using for providing food is actually fostering hunger around the world.

Maintaining a vegan diet is one way that you can help ease the world's burden that is caused by our dependence on animal products. Veganism is thought to be an expensive way of eating. Certainly, it can be very expensive if you eat all the substitute products, but it can be cheap if you buy in bulk and prepare all of your own meals. The reason that eating meat and dairy is so cheap is because the government subsidizes that industry. If the government didn't subsidize meat and dairy, you wouldn't be able to afford them. Market Watch says, "There are estimates out there stating that the price of a single unsubsidized hamburger would cost a whopping $200!" Making meat so cheap isn't good for our bodies or the world. Our government's heavy subsidization of meat and dairy actually affects countries all over the world. According to Market Watch, "The United Nations and other organizations report that farm subsidies in rich countries such as the U.S. depress market prices, so much so that they induce poor countries in Africa and elsewhere to import food that local farmers could otherwise produce more efficiently."

DEALING WITH SOCIAL STIGMA & MISCONCEPTIONS

When you first announce to your friends and family that you're going to be undertaking this big life change, you may encounter some doubters along with people who support you. When Ben went vegan, he did encounter a few doubters. It's unavoidable. Those people will always be around.

There are many ways to deal with these types of people. Ben found that the best way to handle them is by keeping your cool and just educating them. People are afraid of what they don't understand, so share your transformation. Don't let your emotions get the best of you. Just remember that this choice is yours and yours alone. You need to be prepared to answer some serious and also some silly questions that people may have. All of the knowledge that you gain can be very helpful when dealing with doubters. If you show them what you're doing and tell them all about the ins and outs of going vegan, it may help to ease the fear that they may be experiencing.

Another reason why some people might not be so kind to you when you make the transition can be because they don't like the fact that you're making a major life change. If you're in a relationship, your partner might be resentful because they might not have the willpower to change themselves or feel that you're moving on from them. With this type of reaction, it's best to just be very open. Tell them why you're making this change in your life, and try to make them feel included in the change. You'll soon become the in-house expert on veganism, so make sure you're ready to talk about the topic with confidence and knowledge.

One of the biggest misconceptions about vegans is that they're small and feeble. This false stereotype likely stems from the perceived "manliness" of meat-eaters and, by extrapolation, if those who consume flesh are burly and bold, then the opposite must be true of vegans, who fall on the other end of the eating spectrum. Just like meat-eaters, vegans and vegetarians come in all shapes and sizes. Actors Woody Harrelson, Forest Whitaker, NFL running back Ricky Williams, and even rock 'n' roll icons like Bryan Adams, Joan Jett, Phil Collins and Sir Paul McCartney are all veg*n, healthy and proud. One of the most decorated Ironman triathletes, Dave Scott, won the World Championships a record six times while following a strict vegetarian diet. Some of the best endurance athletes on the planet are vegans; among them are Rich Roll, Scott Jurek and Brendan Brazier.

A multiple Ultraman and Ironman Triathlon finisher, Rich Roll is an ultra-endurance all-star. Commonly perceived as the gold standard of triathlons, the Ironman Triathlon is composed of a 2.4-mile swim, 112-mile bike and 26.2-mile run, completed in 17 hours or less. The Ultraman ups the ante considerably with a 6.2-mile swim, 260-mile bike and 52.4-mile run held over three days, with a 12-hour-per-day time limit. Roll is a big advocate of the vegan diet and made history by being the first vegan athlete to compete in an Ultraman Triathlon. Having placed sixth and eleventh at Ultraman Triathlons, it's safe to say that not only is Roll an amazing vegan athlete, he's an extremely fast one too.

Scott Jurek is a major figure in the world of ultrarunning. He not only has seven consecutive wins at the Western States 100-Mile Endurance Run to his name, but accomplished all of this on a plant-based diet. Jurek is very open and passionate about his vegan lifestyle. In his book *Eat and Run: My Unlikely Journey to Ultramarathon Greatness*, Jurek recounts how veganism literally changed his life and his running, and also offers suggestions for how others can incorporate similar changes into their lifestyle to help improve their athletic performance.

Brendan Brazier is an accomplished multisport athlete as well as a longtime vegan. Brazier was a professional Ironman Triathlete from 1998–2004 and a two-time Canadian 50K Ultramarathon Champion. The author of two successful books on veganism, Brazier might be most well known for his line of vegan nutrition products, Vega Nutrition.

These athletes all push the limits of the human body, and plants power them all. The idea that people need meat to grow muscle and become strong is outdated. In the early 1900s, most meals consisted of meat and potatoes—every meal had meat as the centerpiece. Today, many people still have the mind-set that meat needs to be the center of every meal. Just because meat dominated our plates a hundred years ago doesn't mean that it should today.

There's been a slight shift in the number of vegetarians in the U.S. since 2000. According to the 2000 National Zogby Poll sponsored by the Vegetarian Resource Group, "There are about 4.8 million non-institutionalized vegetarian adults in the United States." As of 2008, the number of U.S. adult vegetarians was 7.3 million, or 3.2 percent of the population.

To perform at the highest levels, athletes must be extremely in tune with their bodies and have clear, laser-like focus. These athletes make extremely important, conscious decisions about the foods and products they buy and use. Vegan athletes have an even higher level of knowledge of foods and the effects on their training and performance. When dealing with all-natural food sources, finding the healthiest nutrition to fuel their body is paramount and requires planning and research to ensure their body receives the proper nutrients to accomplish their goals. Practicing veganism opens up a wealth of knowledge about nutrition while providing the natural, healthy ingredients for each athlete to sample and test to develop their own optimal intake devoid of fillers, by-products, hormones and chemicals.

Vegan athletes are strong, resilient, mentally tough and resourceful. These traits are very important as there's always more than one way to accomplish something. This mainly pertains to food, but can obviously be used in other facets of life. Being resourceful as a vegan comes in handy in many situations where animal-free products aren't plentiful. If you're adaptive and creative, you can make something that will satisfy you.

Over time veganism will become more than just a diet. Being vegan should be a source of pride for whomever is making that life choice.

ATHLETIC PERFORMANCE & THE VEGAN LIFESTYLE

The food you eat and your athletic performance go hand in hand. You can work out all day and train hard, but if you're fueling yourself incorrectly, you may be wasting your time. When we think about eating healthy and taking care of our bodies, we always compare ourselves to a Ferrari.

When you're born, you're a like a brand-new sports car: You're in perfect working condition, all your parts mesh seamlessly together with no wear and tear—you even have that new-car (OK, baby) smell! As you get older, maintaining that Ferrari involves "necessary maintenance," in this case eating healthy foods and exercising. Any proud Ferrari owner would put the best fuel in it, wash and wax it constantly, and keep it in pristine condition, right? Think of your body as even more important than a car—you only have this one body with no chance of a trade-in, so you better give it the best care you possibly can.

As a vegan athlete, Ben realized early on that eating a balanced diet is key to maintaining a high level of performance; proper nutrition is even more important than that of some of his fellow competitors and trainees. Since many aspiring vegans who are new to cooking perceive there are limitations of the vegan diet, they can easily fall into the cycle of eating lots of bread and other less-healthy replacement products. These foods can be part of a healthy diet, but they can't be the centerpiece of any balanced diet.

One thing to remember is that not all bodies are created equally. Just because something works well for your friend doesn't mean it'll work well for you. As a vegan, Ben did a lot of experimentation with the food that he ate. You need to try lots of different foods in the early phase of your training to figure out what works best. For some people, a banana might be the superfood that makes them feel superhuman before an event. For others, that same banana can be poison. Experimenting and finding out what works best for you is the a big factor when it comes to performing at a high level.

You can take choosing foods that are right for you to another level entirely by choosing foods that work with your genetic makeup. The Antigen Leukocyte Cellular Antibody Test (ALCAT) is designed to see how your white blood cells react to the foods that you're eating. The test also shows your body's immune response to the foods that you ingested. This may be out of the question for most people, but it just shows the highest level of creating a balanced diet.

Weight Management

Here's a quick quiz: What's more fattening to your body, 3600 calories' worth of vegetables or 3600 calories' worth of peanut butter? Hopefully, you've already realized the answer is "they're both equal in caloric density, therefore they're equally as fattening."

Generally speaking, all calories are the same when it comes to maintaining body weight; the more you take in and the less you burn off, the more weight you'll gain. Of course, there are a plethora of nuances we could go into relating to good calories versus bad calories and very specific nutritional needs in targeted applications, but we're using the most watered-down description for this analogy to talk about portion control for weight management and how serving size can affect the waistline of even the healthiest of vegans.

Just because a tasty sauce, dessert or even your favorite fruit is vegan doesn't mean it's low-calorie and should be consumed en masse. Quite often we've read versions of the phrase "load your plate with all the vegetables you can eat and you won't get fat," and for the most part they're correct—even a huge helping of vegetables won't provide a glut of calories before you're too full to consume any more. Every other vegan food … well, not so much. A vegan cook's repertoire is pretty wide open to some very nutrient- and calorie-rich items, so it's equally as important for vegans to watch their portion control as it is for those practicing less-healthy diets.

Some athletes have an especially difficult time maintaining their energy and weight while training heavily as they can burn an incredible amount of calories, deplete fat and even catabolize muscle. In order to keep a stable weight-to-muscle ratio and high energy levels, it's important to eat several meals throughout the day with the right balance of proteins, carbs and healthy fats to allow for high-level athletic training and racing.

Meal Timing

Developing your own optimal nutritional schedule is not all that different from that of non-vegans and will require some experimentation and practice to get it dialed in to your particular goals and lifestyle. Often when life gets hectic, we don't focus enough on eating properly at specific times throughout the day, yet eating on a structured schedule is one controllable element to maintaining good health.

Most modern nutritional guidelines state that individuals should eat every two to three hours, with small snacks in between. This adds up to five to six meals over the course of a day. This is a good example of adapting to a healthy, structured routine that works for a great deal of people. This smaller meal and snack cadence will also help to keep you full and limit the chances of binge eating later on in the day as your blood sugar and energy reserves fluctuate.

We've found that it works best to eat a majority of our daily caloric intake early in the day with a large breakfast and then eat a nutritious snack every few hours throughout the rest of the day. This plan may not work for everyone, but after having tested multiple different methods of meal timing over the course of the last few years, we've determined without a doubt that it works well for us.

Remember, it's your body and your diet, so research, plan and have fun experimenting to figure out which eating pattern fits your lifestyle and makes you feel the best.

Tip: When the clock strikes noon and everyone from the office wants to head out to grab a bite, this doesn't mean it has to be your lunchtime too. Break the mold by bringing healthy vegan snacks and veggies to eat throughout the day; when your co-workers come back lethargic after a big lunch, you'll still be buzzing along with your glycogen stores topped off properly.

Grocery Shopping

If you primarily stick to buying whole foods, grocery shopping becomes a lot easier, quicker and a lot healthier too. When shopping, keep to the outer perimeter of the store because that's where most of the fresh produce and other whole foods will be. Be sure to read labels while perusing the aisles; don't assume that just because something looks vegan means that it is.

These days, most generic grocery stores will have organic and/or veg*n sections of the store, so if you're looking for veg*n-oriented specialty products, this is where you'll want to start. Also, don't forget about natural and organic grocery store chains, smaller health food stores and online shopping resources. While fresh is best, frozen produce is a good second choice because it's typically picked and frozen at the peak of freshness, thus much of its nutritional value has been preserved.

GENERAL DIETARY NEEDS OF THE VEGAN ATHLETE

Whether you're intent on gaining muscle or losing weight, you still need to consume fat, protein and carbohydrates to provide your body with the necessary fuel to sustain life and systemic function. In this area, a vegan athlete is no different than someone who chooses to eat animal proteins. The healthy, natural sources a vegan uses to get these important vitamins, minerals and building blocks of proper nutrition are unique.

If you're new to a vegan diet or are a practicing vegan who's new to exercise, you should be aware of your fat, protein and carbohydrate intake in order to maintain a healthy physique with plenty of energy to function at high intensities. You should also take stock of the vital components needed for making hormones, muscles and other essential biological equipment.

Protein

Composed of amino acids, this essential nutrient is required by the body for cellular growth and maintenance. Abundant in muscles, protein can be found in all cells of the body and is a major structural component of all organs, hair and skin. The amino acids that provide the building blocks for protein are responsible for creating new tissue and repairing damaged tissue, especially muscles. Ingesting protein from food is extremely important and provides nine essential amino acids that aren't synthesized by the body.

Protein deficiency can lead to a variety of ailments, fatigue and hair or muscle loss. An early warning sign of protein deficiency is a drop in energy and an overall lack of motivation and malaise. Most veg*ns will experience higher than normal energy levels when converting to a wholly plant-based diet, so any sudden drop in energy should be an indication that you may not be ingesting enough protein in your diet.

When someone makes the change from the standard American diet (SAD) to a vegan diet, one of the first concerns is usually getting enough protein to maintain or build muscle. Copious amounts of protein from animal flesh are extremely common in the SAD diet, while vegans must find their sources of (leaner, healthier) proteins from vegetables, nuts and legumes. Contrary to popular belief, plant-based diets can be extremely high in protein thanks to the myriad of choices featuring essential amino acids. Don't believe us? Check out "2 Weeks to Eat Like a Vegan" on page 50 for dozens of different delicious items that'll help you get the proper levels of proteins along with heart-healthy fats and energy-boosting carbs.

In an effort to go vegan, some individuals remove the animal-based proteins from their diet and rely on bread, pasta and other carbohydrate-filled foods to keep them satiated—to the detriment of their waistline and overall health. Just cutting out meats alone doesn't give you free reign to overdo any other food group, especially carbs. While carbohydrates are essential for producing energy, excess carbs are easily converted to fat and stored in the body. Relying too much on carb-heavy foods like bread and pasta is a sure way to pack on additional weight even when cutting out animal flesh from your diet.

Plant or Animal Proteins: Which Is Better?

"Better" is a relative term because both plant- and animal-based proteins have their own benefits. Protein is more abundant in animal flesh than it is in an equal-sized serving of any plant-based food. For example, it'd take approximately 2 cups of lentils to provide the same amount of protein found in 3.5 ounces of chicken breast. This comparison doesn't really hold much weight, however, as a well-rounded plant-based diet consists of many different menu items that contain protein: veggies, beans, grains, tofu, nut butter, soy milk, brown rice and more. Plant-based proteins are far superior to those found in animal flesh because they don't have the saturated fat and cholesterol common in meat-based protein; they're also lower in calories. For a lean, healthy, athletic physique, plant-based proteins provide all the benefits of high-quality building blocks of life without any of the adverse health effects of eating animal flesh.

How Much Protein Do You Need?

A sedentary individual should consume about 0.37 grams of protein per day for every pound of body weight. (For example, a 150-pound male would need about 5.5 grams of protein in a 24-hour period.) Active people should consume .5 to .75 grams of protein per day based on their body weight. Athletes who train regularly should increase their protein consumption to 1 to 1.5 grams of protein per day for every pound of body weight. The highest end of the scale is usually reserved for athletes looking to gain or maintain a large amount of muscle mass.

Delicious and nutritious sources of vegan protein include legumes, brown and wild rice, nuts and soy products. A simple high-protein vegan snack could be soy yogurt with a handful of almonds thrown in. When focusing on eating a balanced vegan diet, it's not very difficult to get the recommended daily amount of protein to maintain healthy, lean muscle mass.

The Soy Question: How Much is Too Much?

Providing all of the amino acids essential to human nutrition and body function, soy seems like it's the perfect addition to a veg*n diet to replace animal-based protein. Pound for pound in tofu, soy contains nearly the same amount of protein as animal flesh and can be cooked in myriad ways with countless different flavors; it even can be made into foods that would fool a meat-eater. Unfortunately, the jury is still out on the health risks of eating too much soy, specifically the effects on estrogen levels that may be a precursor for developing breast cancer and whether soy has a negative effect on the thyroid.

While there are no concrete answers and plenty of smoking guns revealed as of this printing, the judicious and responsible answer is to limit the amount of soy products in your diet until further studies have been concluded and you can make an educated decision for yourself. Eating tofu two to three times a week, a daily 8-ounce glass of soy milk or a few serving of tempeh, miso or edamame a week should not be detrimental to your health at all. If you have any questions about your soy consumption and the associated risks, please contact your doctor.

Iron

Necessary for the transport of oxygen in the blood, iron is extremely important for proper circulatory function. Plants contain a significant amount of iron, albeit in the non-heme form, which is more sensitive to inhibitors than protein from animal flesh. Iron-rich foods should be consumed with vitamin C as it helps to convert iron into something that's more bioavailable (or usable) by the body. A simple trick to get more iron into your body is by cooking your vegan meals in a new cast-iron skillet; as your food cooks, the iron from the skillet with get absorbed into it.

Note: Refrain from cooking food for children under the age of three in iron skillets as it can cause iron toxicity. Dried beans, dark leafy vegetables such as spinach and broccoli, black and pinto beans, and cashews and almonds are great vegan sources of iron.

Vitamin B12

Playing a vital role in the proper functioning of the brain and nervous system, B12 is also the largest and most structurally complicated vitamin needed by the human body. This water-soluble vitamin doesn't exist naturally in non-animal-based foods, therefore vegans and vegetarians should look for B12-fortified foods (such as certain soy milks and cereals) to supplement what they lack. A vitamin B12 deficiency in the short-term is responsible for fatigue or depression; in severe cases it can lead to irreversible damage to the central nervous system and brain.

Calcium

Required for strong bones and healthy teeth, calcium is abundant in several items common to a plant-based diet. Dark green, leafy vegetables, tofu and calcium-fortified non-dairy milk are often mentioned as excellent sources for veg*ns to obtain their daily calcium intake needs, recommended at 1000mg per day. A common misconception is that veg*ns tend to be deficient in calcium, but recent research has uncovered evidence that the opposite is true—animal proteins are responsible for leaching calcium from bones while plant-based proteins don't result in the same reduction in calcium content and bone density. Almonds, broccoli and tahini are also recommended sources for maintaining a diet with the proper amount of calcium.

Carbohydrates

Used by the human body as a primary source of energy, carbohydrates are simple or complex sugars that are broken down into glucose within the body. Simple carbohydrates are sugars made of one or two molecules that are easily absorbed into the bloodstream and are responsible for rapid, short-term energy boosts. White and brown sugar, honey, corn syrup, jams, jellies and most fruit drinks and soft drinks fall into this category and provide little nutrient benefit other than energy from calories. Most often associated with sweets and candies, simple carbs are often attributed to weight gain from empty calories and a spike in energy followed by a crash of lethargy.

For endurance athletes, energy gels and carb-loaded drinks used during extreme training and racing provide a necessary dose of energy during long and grueling events. If an athlete doesn't have the proper amount of glucose, his performance will diminish rapidly as his energy stores are depleted. This eventually leads to the dreaded "bonk" when his body just quits. The average individual can do just fine without ingesting too many simple carbs as they do little for health benefits but can significantly add to their waistline over time.

Complex carbs are found in green vegetables, whole-grain breads, oatmeal, beans, lentils and peas, as well as starchy vegetables such as potatoes, sweet corn and pumpkin. These sources provide a slower-digesting source of carbs to keep blood sugar levels more stable and avoid the spikes and valleys of simple sugars. Since complex carbs are found in whole foods, they are also excellent sources for other vitamins and minerals and make up part of a healthy diet.

With the prevailing thought that "carbs are bad" currently swirling around dieting fads, it's important to distinguish between carbs. Complex carbs such as green leafy vegetables, whole-grain breads, oatmeal, beans and sweet potatoes are not the enemy. Simple carbs (or, shall we say, sugars) found in soft drinks, fruit juices, candy, white bread and white flour pastas are the ones healthy individuals should strive to avoid or only indulge in occasionally.

Whole grains

Whole grains are just that—entire grains that haven't had their outer covering removed. When something is listed as having whole grains, this means that all three parts of the grain were used: bran, endosperm and germ. The bran is the outermost coating of the kernel and makes up less than 15 percent of the kernel. The endosperm is the largest portion by volume of the kernel, at slightly over 80 percent, and is the portion that's normally extracted for use in white flour. Finally, the smallest portion of the kernel is called the germ; it's the part of the seed that sprouts and contains the most protein per gram in the entire kernel.

One thing that most people don't know is that whole grains contain antioxidants that aren't found in some fruits and vegetables. Whole grains are a good source of B vitamins, vitamin E, magnesium, iron and fiber. Most of the antioxidants and vitamins are found in the germ and the bran of a grain. Vitamin E is a strong antioxidant that has the power to protect your body from certain cancer-causing chemicals. Whole grains have been shown to reduce the risk of heart disease by decreasing cholesterol levels, blood pressure and blood coagulation. Some great whole grains to have on hand include brown rice, wild rice, quinoa, whole oats, popcorn and bulgur wheat.

Carbs: How Much Is Right for You?

The U.S. Department of Agriculture indicates that all humans need between 45 and 65 percent of their calories from carbohydrates. Each gram of carbs is worth 4 calories. During training for triathlons, an average triathlete eats about 2600 calories per day; carbohydrates account for about 1600 calories. This means on any given day, they consume approximately 400 grams of carbs. While that may seem like a very high amount, remember that almost every single food that you consume contains carbohydrates in some quantity; fruits, vegetables, grains and nuts are staples of the vegan diet and they all contain carbs. Some other great vegan-friendly sources that'll help you top off your energy stores are raisins, garbanzo beans, prunes, sweet potatoes and bananas.

Fats

The "low-fat" diet craze that persisted throughout the end of the last century still has a tiny foothold on some eaters. The thought that fats make you fat and that low-fat foods are better than full-fat items has been completely disproven, yet take a quick peek at packaged or processed foods in any grocery aisle and you'll see plenty of low-fat alternatives. A quick rule of thumb when you read "low-fat" on the front of product packaging: Just say no. Look at the label on the back and you'll usually see the fat content is slightly lower and the calories are higher—it's not the fat that they take out that's the problem, it's the additional ingredients like sugar that are put in! Of course, we're not bashing all low-fat foods—veggies, fruits and grains are already low in fat and good for you.

Simply put, ingesting fat in moderation does not make you fat. Period. Actually, fat content in food will satiate you for longer periods of time and help prevent cravings to snack in between meals. Monounsaturated and polyunsaturated fats are essential to the human diet as they provide alpha-linoleic acid (omega-3) and linoleic acid (omega-6), which may lower blood pressure, decrease inflammation (thus reducing arthritis), decreasing the risk of a heart attack and stroke, reduce depression, prevent dementia, lower your risk of sudden cardiac death, and even reduce the risk of some types of cancer. A very small amount of saturated fats is beneficial for bone and skin health; less than 5 percent of daily calories are recommended.

Monounsaturated fats are found in olive, canola and sunflower oil, avocados, peanuts, cashews and almonds. Polyunsaturated fats are abundant in flaxseed, safflower oil, walnuts, chia seeds and seaweed. Saturated fats can be found in coconut oil, palm kernel oil, cottonseed oil and chocolate.

All's not completely well in the world of fats, however, as long as trans fats made with hydrogenated or partially hydrogenated oils are in anyone's diet. According to a 2006 scientific review in the *New England Journal of Medicine*: "From a nutritional standpoint, the consumption of trans fatty acids results in considerable potential for harm but no apparent benefit."

That surely doesn't sound like a ringing endorsement! As a vegan, you already sidestep the trans fat that occurs naturally in the meat and milk of cattle and sheep, but you need to remain vigilant for hydrogenated or partially hydrogenated oils in any prepared food you purchase. Veg*ns are especially at risk, as many prepackaged products often contain these potentially harmful fats to replace animal fats. Luckily, regulations, bans and various markings on packaging are in place in most Westernized nations around the world, allowing careful consumers to spot and avoid trans fats.

For healthy adults, the USDA recommends that 20 to 35 percent of your daily calories come from fat. For most individuals that falls between 44 and 77 grams of fat daily. As mentioned above, the sources should be a balance of polyunsaturated and monounsaturated fats, along with a very small amount of saturated fats.

Vegan Staples

To make eating easier, make sure to have your home stocked with quick and healthy options. Some staple foods that you should always have include:

Nuts

These can usually be found in the bulk section of your supermarket. When buying them, look for raw, unsalted nuts. Raw nuts usually don't have hydrogenated oils on them like roasted nuts do. Hydrogenated oils aren't natural and our bodies can't efficiently process them like healthy olive, canola, flaxseed, sunflower, safflower or vegetable oils. Hydrogenated and partially hydrogenated oils are known as "trans fat" and have been linked to diabetes, cancer and cardiovascular disease. Due to the health risks, most European countries have banned its use in foods.

A great source of protein as well as vitamins, minerals and fiber, nuts are also high in essential omega-3 and omega-6 fatty acids, amino acids that are vital for cell repair and production. Nuts pack a high-calorie density into a small form factor, and can be a great snack to satiate a growling tummy between meals. However, they can also be responsible for adding some additional belly real estate if overeaten. Walnuts, cashews, macadamia nuts and almonds can pack about 400 calories per 2.5-ounce portions, and while they're providing protein and many important vitamins like folate, copper, manganese, B12, magnesium and vitamin E, you shouldn't go overboard if you're trying to keep a close eye on your calorie intake. A handful of nuts twice a day is a great, moderate snack for the healthy vegan.

Fruits & Vegetables

As a vegan, Ben appreciates all the color that he gets to eat on a daily basis. You can never have enough fruits and vegetables around—go ahead and pig out on them. Although fruit is great for you, you can't survive on fruit alone. Vegetables need to be incorporated as well into a healthy diet. When you're eating fruits and vegetables, make sure that you balance out all the sweet fruit with more bitter vegetables. Fruits are rich in simple carbohydrates but they contain very little protein, complex carbohydrates and healthy fats, all of which are essential nutrients. Vegetables provide complex carbohydrates, healthy fats and proteins and are extremely well suited to give your body the vitamins and minerals needed as well as maintain a steady supply of slow-burning sugars to keep your blood sugar balanced throughout the day.

TIP: To maximize a quick shot of healthy energy from fruit, consume it on an empty stomach. Fruit contains simple sugars that quickly enter the bloodstream, and they won't stay in the stomach for very long. When fruit is eaten with other foods, it doesn't get broken down nearly as efficiently as it does by itself.

TIP: Fruit is a great post-workout food since it contains a high amount of water to rehydrate our bodies after a tough workout. Fruit is also filled with carbohydrates, which our bodies convert into glucose to use for fuel.

Veg*n Superfoods

It's a bird, it's a plane ... well, maybe not. The term "superfood" seems to be used all over the place. Goji berries, açaí berries, blueberries and any combination of natural(ish) foods with antioxidants get this word plastered across their labels. Testimonials and infomercials aside, the amount of antioxidants in most of these products make such a small difference in the magnitude of free radicals in your system you'd be hard-pressed to call them "super"; they'd be more aptly called "quite good, delicious and slightly helpful foods," but somehow that's just not as good for marketing purposes.

Have no fear, though—there really are some foods that have all the characteristics you'd want in a prolific wonder-food; vitamins, minerals, protein, fiber, slow-burning carbohydrates and healthy fats. Some of these real edible superheroes are quinoa, chia, flax and coconut oil, and you'll find them included in the recipes located in the appendix.

Quinoa (pronounced *keen-wah*) closely resembles a grain (although it's more closely related to spinach than wheat), is gluten-free and contains a high protein content, fiber, phosphorous, magnesium, iron and calcium. For vegans, the combination of iron, protein and calcium makes it extremely beneficial to add to their diets in place of the less nutrient-dense rice or couscous. Quinoa is also very versatile and can be made into a protein-packed breakfast cereal with fruit, berries and nuts, a great cold salad with tofu, corn, beans and chopped onions, and complements nearly any meal as a healthy, filling and delicious side dish. Check out the recipes in the appendix starting on page 90 for more examples of putting this superfood to work in your meals.

Chia is both mythical in its origin and usage and almost, well, a bit of a joke. Referring to the latter, chia is the sprout that grows out of some of the most unusually shaped herb gardens. Yes, we're referring to Chia Pets. Who would've thought the humorous plant filling out the mohawk in a Mr. T Chia Pet would be an amazingly healthy food that has followers believing it provides superhuman strength and endurance? After all, in *Born to Run* by Christopher McDougall, the Tarahumara Indians claim a tablespoon of chia seeds is all the fuel a grown man would need to run for 24 hours or 50 to 100 miles on some of the incredibly challenging trails in the Copper Canyons. A part of the Aztec warrior's diet, chia seeds pack protein, fiber, omega-3 fatty acids, antioxidants, calcium, phosphorus, magnesium, manganese, copper, iron, molybdenum, niacin and zinc into a very small package. One of the neatest things about chia is how it can be prepared into a vitamin-packed energy drink: simply stir a tablespoon of dry chia seeds into a 10-ounce glass of water with a spritz of lime or lemon and wait a few minutes. As the seeds soak in the water, they start to gel and make an unusual syrupy drink with a nutty and citrusy flavor. Add honey, agave or even some fruit juice and stir to taste. Chia seeds are also great when sprinkled on oatmeal or baked in bread.

Flaxseeds are fantastic sources of healthy fat, fiber, protein, an abundance of micronutrients and omega-3 fatty acids. There's even some evidence that they may help reduce your risk of heart disease, cancer, stroke and diabetes. Containing prostaglandins, a potent anti-inflammatory, flaxseeds can help reduce muscle soreness and aid in the process of repairing the microtears in muscle from strenuous exercise. With a slightly nutty flavor akin to wheat germ, flaxseed can be added to cereals, salads, hummus and mashed potatoes, ground up and sprinkled over vegan sorbet, even swirled in a smoothie. In baking, flaxseeds can be a great substitute for eggs, flour or oil in recipes and also provide a distinctive flavor in muffins and breads.

Coconut oil can be a bit of a conundrum for some. It has provided the primary source of fat in the diets of millions of people for generations, yet it's high in saturated fat and thus many agencies worldwide

(FDA, WHO, Dieticians of Canada, etc.) recommended that its consumption be limited. How can this dichotomy exist? The furor started with a 1994 Center for Science in the Public Interest report that partially hydrogenated used to pop movie theater popcorn delivered as much saturated fat as six McDonald's Big Mac burgers. Remember the heart-attack-inducing, arterial villains called "partially hydrogenated oils" from page 39?

Virgin coconut oil that hasn't been hydrogenated still packs a lot of saturated fat, but current research has begun to show that small amounts are not harmful. In fact, supporters of coconut oil purport antibacterial, antimicrobial and antiviral properties in the oil that speed up metabolism, fight acne and even have the potential to cure everything from baldness and asthma to kidney stones and tuberculosis. For a vegan, the benefits of this fiber-, vitamin- and mineral-rich oil also lie in its ability to replace butter and eggs in baking and create flaky pie crusts, crumbly scones, fluffy cupcake icings and more.

FOODS THAT VEGANS SHOULD BE AWARE OF

As you continue on your path toward veganism, you'll develop a higher sense of comfort with the foods you eat. It'll increasingly become more natural and eventually you may even stop reading nutrition labels ... well, not so fast. Even after multiple years of living this lifestyle and being extremely aware of what he's ingesting, Ben still reads all of the nutrition labels of food he's thinking of buying before he makes his purchase. He's learned the hard way that just because a particular food appears to be vegan doesn't always mean that it is. Here are a few "gotchas" that can undermine even the most experienced vegans if they're not aware:

HONEY: Honey is obviously made from bees. Although people have been eating and using honey for thousands of years, strict vegans don't consume honey on the grounds that it's created by bees for bees, not for humans.

BEER: Most beers contain isinglass, which is a fining agent that's used to clarify beer and give it that clear, glossy look. Unfortunately, isinglass is made from the swim bladders of fish–not quite what you'd expect from a frosty cold beer, huh?

NON-DAIRY WHIPPED TOPPINGS: Please note that just because a topping is labeled as "non-dairy" doesn't mean that it's truly dairy-free. That's because most non-dairy whipped toppings commonly found in supermarkets contain casein (in the form of sodium caseinate), which is a milk protein derivative. So be sure to carefully read the labels and be on the lookout for this.

DRY-ROASTED NUTS: Not all dry-roasted nuts are not vegan, but some of the bigger-name brands use gelatin to help keep the coating on the nuts. And that brings us to:

ANYTHING WITH GELATIN IN IT: Gelatin is made from the ground-up connective tissue (e.g., skin, cartilage, tendons) and bones of animals (particularly cows, chicken, horses and pigs), and is hidden in everything from Jell-O, marshmallows, gummy bears and most chewy candies to jellies and jams.

SEAWEED: Even though it's a plant, seaweed isn't vegan because it typically contains bits of fish matter and crustaceans.

Want to learn more about what brands or restaurants are vegan-friendly? Get on the Internet and do a little research. PETA provides an up-to-date resource for researching brands, foods and restaurants. If you prefer going mobile, download one of the many apps available for your smartphone to help you make educated choices.

Vegan To-Go

Traveling and keeping a vegan diet used to be a hassle, but over the last few years the number of vegans around the world has exploded. The result? Many more choices at restaurants and grocery stores. You can also plan ahead and take your own food!

When traveling, pack foods that are small and compact, like granola bars or pre-cut fruit packets. Most airports sell some type of vegan trail mix blend or maybe even a vegan protein bar. Chances are you can probably find a prepackaged salad as well. Some airlines even offer vegan-friendly in-flight meals; make sure to inquire about it before your flight. With a little research before your travels, you can easily have everything handled. If you have a smartphone, use it to find vegan-friendly restaurants in a new area.

When traveling for long distances, it's easiest to pack things that don't require refrigeration. Non-perishable snacks like kale chips, granola, oven-roasted edamame, nuts and dried fruit are all good examples. Keep them readily accessible.

FUELING FOR TRAINING & EVENTS

Sports nutrition for athletes is complicated, to say the least. Figuring out what foods work best for any athlete takes some time and experimentation. Being a vegan doesn't make this process much easier, but it does have one incredible advantage to a standard diet: Since all the foods you'll be eating are from natural sources, you can dial in your nutrition without having to worry about artificial ingredients, hormones or other chemicals that can disrupt your body's systems and hamper your performance.

This is yet another reason why the number of plant-fueled athletes seems to be rising every day. To service this growing market, more companies are creating vegan-friendly products. "Vegan sports nutrition" has actually become a growing market, although some of the products can be quite pricey.

If you can't find vegan sports nutrition or simply can't afford them, the preferred method is to use real, natural food to fuel your body. What we mean by "real food" is that you make it yourself—it's not prepackaged. A lot of the "health" foods that are being pushed on athletes are actually not much better than your standard candy bar. Training with real food works well because it can be perfectly tailored to what your tastes and needs so you can discover what works well for you.

Race-Day Foods

After months of training, sacrifices and preparation, race day has finally arrived and the most important fueling of your body is about to take place. Although each individual athlete's palate and nutritional requirements are different, a common rule of thumb is to increase carbohydrate intake for three to six days leading up to an endurance event; on race morning consume a meal that'll provide you with some slow-burning carbs for prolonged energy along with a bit of fat and protein to maintain satiety and act as a backup source of energy once the initial blood glycogen dips due to exerted effort. It's important for this meal to be light on the stomach as running, biking, swimming and most vigorous activities will not only make a full belly feel uncomfortable, your body will be forced to divert blood flow to your stomach to aid in digestion. Here are a couple examples of light, quick and effective meals/snacks that'll provide the energy to start an event off right.

FROZEN FRUIT: This is a staple in all our events and training. As stated earlier in the book, fruit is a great food to keep you full and energized. All you do is slice up some fruit and freeze it overnight. When you begin training, you can just leave the frozen bag of fruit in your jersey or wherever else you store your nutrition. It'll defrost as you train and be nice and cold when you're ready to eat it.

PEANUT BUTTER AND BANANA SANDWICHES: With a great balance of protein and carbs as well as some potassium from the bananas, P&B sandwiches are also light enough on the stomach to eat about an hour before training or an event as well as provide a great recovery meal.

Pre-Race Hydration

Hydrating for training or events is not much different for a vegan than it is for any other athlete. Your body needs liquids along with proper minerals and nutrients to keep it functioning and to keep you in motion.

Luckily, a great deal of hydration products are vegan, so it's not that difficult to find something that will suit your needs. To maximize your ability to be fully hydrated, you should start consuming a 3:1 mix of water to electrolyte sports drink a few days prior to any big training day or race. Starting the hydration process a few days before your event or training will allow your cells adequate time to absorb the maximum amount of life-sustaining water. Also, the plant-based vegan diet will help a great deal as these foods contain a high water content that will also help to hydrate your body. Fruits and vegetables not only hydrate your body, they provide plenty of the vitamins and minerals that your body needs.

Post-Race Recovery

For post-exercise recovery and inflammation reduction, eating foods rich in omega-3 fatty acids, protein, carbohydrates, zinc, magnesium and some antioxidants within the first half hour after a workout is recommended. A 4:1 carb-to-protein ratio is optimal for refueling and repairing muscle tissue.

Omega-3 fatty acids found in flaxseeds, chia seeds, walnuts, avocados, raspberries, soy and kidney beans contain anti-inflammatory compounds called prostaglandins that help to heal the microtears formed in muscles from strenuous exercise. Protein has been shown to reduce exercise-induced muscle damage, which is caused in part by inflammation. Antioxidants, like those found in green tea and red/purple/blue berries, can help minimize inflammation and oxidative stress because they abolish free radicals and inhibit the production of enzymes that cause irritation and pain. Lastly, carbohydrates are used to replenish your depleted glycogen stores.

THE BEGINNER'S 3-STEP GUIDE TO GOING VEGAN

Are you ready to embrace a healthier, less wasteful and less environmentally destructive nutritional lifestyle? Even if you aren't currently on board with the socioeconomic reasons involved with the entire vegan lifestyle, you can become a vegan and develop natural eating habits that'll have the possibility to improve your health and increase your longevity. Many vegans report feeling healthier, more energized, more in tune with their bodies and more connected to the foods they eat and their environment within days or weeks of making the switch. For some, the change is monumental and life-altering. Others can view it as a nutritional choice based on solid science and environmental factors—removing the impurities, diseases and biotoxins that can be found in animal flesh constitutes a choice in healthier eating options for them and their families.

Once you're ready to give going vegan a try, here's an extremely basic 3-Step Guide to Going Vegan. With this, or any nutritional program, it's important that you speak to your doctor to find out if you have any health conditions that may not respond well to any new type of diet. Making the switch is as difficult as you make it out to be—choose a less stressful time of life to make this transformation and focus on your goals to give yourself the drive to follow through.

Step 1: Write down your reasons for wanting to maintain a vegan diet.

This is the most important step. You need to have concrete reasons for why you want to change your eating habits and lifestyle. Without a few solid reasons to do this, you will not be able to complete the transition successfully. Your reasons can be anything, it is just important to have something that drives you. Some of the more popular reasons include: the health benefits, animal welfare, environmental protection or moral reasons. The reason can be all yours; do not worry about what people think. This decision does not affect anyone other than you. Luckily for you, this book covers most of the important steps to becoming vegan.

TIP: Keep it simple! You don't need to be a world-class chef like Corey Irwin in order to be vegan. With fruit and vegetables on hand, you can whip up plenty of meals that take no time at all.

This book will provide you with all the information you will need to make the transformation to your new healthy vegan lifestyle. We did the research for you!

Use *The Vegan Athlete* to learn:

- Which foods you should eat
- Which you shouldn't eat
- The impact that eating animal products has on your body and the environment
- Which vitamins or supplements you should include in your diet
- Simple recipes
- Which books to read, podcasts to listen to or smartphone apps to get (this is a stage that should never have an end; you should be constantly looking up new recipes and information about veganism)

Step 2: Set small goals.

Now that you've figured out your reasons for going vegan and done some research, it's time to set some small goals. One way to help you in setting your goals would be to keep a small food journal for a week. Once you've taken a look at what you eat, it's time to start the vegan journey. Perhaps the easiest and most pain-free way to transition is to slowly remove things by setting goals. After looking at your journal, you can pick something non-vegan to get rid of. Here's an example:

Week 1: You notice that you drink a lot of milk, so for week one your goal could be to cut out milk from your diet. You can simply stop using milk in your coffee, cereal or wherever else you use it. For the sake of keeping it simple, don't worry about whether dairy is an ingredient in the foods you eat. If you eat a lot of cereal and think that it can't be done without milk, you'd be mistaken. There are plenty of delicious nut- and plant-based milks made of almond, cashew, hazelnut, hemp or soy that work wonderfully. Just take it slowly!

Week 2: Continue abstaining from whatever you dropped from your diet in week one and add one more thing. Also, now that you've stopped drinking dairy in the last week, you can start eliminating dairy from foods that you eat as well. So that means you can't eat any food that contains dairy. All you need to do is look at the ingredient list.

TIP: You're not alone: Most people's bodies crave the "Three S's": salty, savory and sweet. Don't worry, there are plenty of options for you to easily find all of these flavors in a plant-based diet so you won't feel deprived.

If you aren't the most kitchen-savvy person, planning out a few simple vegan meals for the first week or two can make the transition even easier since this takes all of the guesswork out of eating.

Step 3: Begin your vegan lifestyle.

Now that you have all of this great information about your diet and veganism, it's time to put it into practice. If you slip up over the first few weeks, don't dwell on it—just move on and learn from your mistake. Your body will appreciate your new clean diet.

We've even provided some resources to make it even easier for you. Starting on page 90 you can find easy recipes for delicious vegan meals, desserts, snacks and drinks that show that eating healthy and earth consciously doesn't have to be bland or boring! The Great Vegan Swap on page 115 makes it easy for you to substitute vegan ingredients in any other recipe so you can make the meals you enjoy even healthier. Finally, we list vegan resources that are so helpful for articles, research, recipes and insight and reflection on living the vegan lifestyle.

2 WEEKS TO EAT LIKE A VEGAN

We've already debunked the "there are so few choices as a vegan, there's nothing to eat" myth, but with Corey Irwin's help we're going to make it even simpler for you to find healthy, tasty and nutritious vegan meals, drinks and snacks. No, it's not the same thing every day. These menu choices don't repeat and there are hundreds of different foods that make up millions of different meal combinations.

To help you begin your vegan lifestyle, here's a two-week meal plan with simple, easy-to-prepare meals and snacks. You'll find many of the recipes in the appendix. Not a gourmet chef? Did the last recipe you read have something to do with opening a lemonade stand in grade school? Well, don't worry—many of the items in the two-week plan are as simple as peeling a banana or slicing up a bell pepper. Vegan cooking is actually simpler in many areas than preparing traditional food as you can rule out the fears of cooking a meat to the proper temperature in order to kill off bacteria or other pathogens. For the most part, you'll just be dealing with ingredients that should be washed thoroughly prior to preparation. The instructions for the recipes, which Corey Irwin expressly created for this book, were purposely written to give you the guidance and support you need to be more productive and confident in the kitchen.

Week 1

	Breakfast	Snack	Lunch	Snack	Dinner	Snack
Monday	A bowl of oatmeal with fresh fruit, honey and coconut milk, accompanied by a cup of green tea	Baked eggplant and zucchini slices covered with shredded vegan cheese, panko bread crumbs, sea salt and olive oil	Southwestern Black Bean Salsa Tortilla Wrap (page 92)	Banana and a handful of almonds	Marinated grilled mushroom, red onion, green and red bell pepper, and tofu skewers (baste in store-bought vegan marinade)	Air-popped popcorn with a dash of garlic salt and olive oil

TIP: You may have noticed that we included an after-dinner snack. If your body's hungry, eat. Listen to your body!

	Breakfast	Snack	Lunch	Snack	Dinner	Snack
Tuesday	Two slices of whole-grain toast spread with nut butter, maple syrup and microwaved apricot (or peach) slices, sprinkled with cinnamon	Frozen grapes	Tomato, avocado, cucumber and sprout sandwich spread with store-bought hummus	Potato and steamed broccoli topped with vegan cheese	Chana Masala (page 95) with Aromatic Basmati Rice (page 102)	Scoop of chocolate soy ice cream topped with fresh red raspberries and crushed hazelnuts
Wednesday	"Blueberry Blast" Breakfast Smoothie (page 97)	Sliced ripe plantains with vanilla soy yogurt	Cucumber, Tomato and Artichoke Salad (page 106) with a side of pita chips and store-bought roasted red bell pepper dip	A handful of store-bought tamari nuts	Store-bought spinach and soy cheese whole wheat vegan pizza with a small side salad	Microwaved baked apple with cinnamon, dried cherries and chopped walnuts

TIP: If you have a hard time eating food in the morning, try smoothies instead. Smoothies are easy on your digestive system and provide easily digestible calories and nutrients.

	Breakfast	Snack	Lunch	Snack	Dinner	Snack
Thursday	Whole wheat bagel with vegan cheese spread and tomato slice	Red bell pepper slices with store-bought tapenade	Nut butter and banana sandwich served with store-bought baked veggie chips on the side	Toasted pita topped with olive oil, dried oregano and thyme leaves, and sea salt	Chinese Eggplant and Tofu Stir-Fry (page 94)	Apricot-Papaya Pudding Parfait (page 114)

TIP: You can easily get away with a big breakfast so don't worry too much about calories. This doesn't mean you can eat donuts, though. As the day progresses, your meals should become smaller and lighter due to your lower caloric expenditure as the day comes to a close.

	Breakfast	Snack	Lunch	Snack	Dinner	Snack
Friday	Whole-grain (dry) cereal with soy milk and nectarine slices	Pineapple, kiwi and starfruit slices with coconut milk	Mexican-Style Gazpacho (page 107), served with store-bought vegan pinto bean spread on a crusty slice of toasted bread	Steamed butternut squash topped with melted vegan cheese	Mushroom-Olive Quinoa Pilaf with Fresh Herbs (page 91), served with a side salad of romaine hearts, walnuts, pears and beets, drizzled with balsamic vinaigrette	Mango Pie with Cardamom and Saffron (page 110)

Week 1

	Breakfast	Snack	Lunch	Snack	Dinner	Snack
Saturday	Mushroom and soy cheese omelet made with egg substitute, served with a small bowl of red raspberries and blackberries	Store-bought baba ghanoush on crackers, topped with Kalamata olives	Steamed kale with avocados, scallions, chickpeas and grape tomatoes, seasoned with sea salt, lemon juice, olive oil and black pepper	Handful of pumpkin seeds mixed with dried fruit (apricots, raisins, etc.)	Penne with Cashew-Walnut Pesto and Sun-Dried Tomatoes (page 96)	Vegan chocolate–covered banana slices (use a fork to dip banana slices into a mug of microwaved chocolate and then cool on a plate)

TIP: If you think you need a ton of cooking equipment to make all of this food, you're wrong! All of these recipes can be done using two pots, a pan, one large mixing bowl and a utensil or two.

	Breakfast	Snack	Lunch	Snack	Dinner	Snack
Sunday	Watermelon-Coconut Sports Recovery Drink (page 97)	Cucumber slices topped with store-bought sundried tomato spread	Store-bought roasted tomato and basil soup (from a carton), served with strawberry and spinach salad topped with pistachios and sherry vinaigrette	Granola bar	Spaghetti squash topped with tomato sauce and vegan cheese	Raw Asian pear slices spread with almond butter and drizzled with honey (or maple syrup)

TIP: Many big-name-brand granola bars aren't vegan so make sure to read the ingredient list before purchasing. You can easily find a vegan granola or energy bar at any major supermarket.

Week 2

	Breakfast	Snack	Lunch	Snack	Dinner	Snack
Monday	Store-bought, no-sugar-added muesli served with soy milk	Dry-roasted edamame sprinkled with olive oil, sea salt and black pepper	Steamed spinach topped with sunflower seeds, served with a glass of lemon water	Dried mango slices	Roasted beets with toasted walnuts, thyme, garlic, olive oil, lemon juice, salt and pepper	Frozen banana "custard" (put frozen banana in food processor and pulse until just combined)

Week 2

	Breakfast	Snack	Lunch	Snack	Dinner	Snack
Tuesday	Kasha (buckwheat) porridge with almond milk and fresh fruit, served with a cup of Unbelievably Creamy and Delicious, "I-Can't-Believe-It's-Vegan," All Natural, Hot and Spicy, Sugar-Free Cocoa (page 98)	Store-bought salsa, guacamole and baked tortilla chips topped with melted vegan cheese	Store-bought butternut squash soup (from a carton) with a piece of crusty Kalamata olive bread	Cut-up veggies and store-bought vegan white bean dip	Acorn squash drizzled with maple syrup and seasoned with a pinch of nutmeg, served with chickpea, cucumber, red onion and mint side salad	A glass of Niña Colada Punch (page 100)
Wednesday	Peanut butter–banana smoothie (combine frozen banana chunks and peanut butter in a blender)	A handful of toasted almonds and dried cherries	Asian-style noodles, julienned jicama, sliced almonds and red bell pepper, marinated in a store-bought soy-ginger dressing	Baked egg in an avocado, topped with freshly squeezed lemon juice, salt and pepper	Seasoned and steamed zucchini, yellow squash, tomatoes and white beans, served with a side of wild rice pilaf	Pear and Apple Crisp (page 109) with a cup of green tea
Thursday	Cantaloupe topped with red raspberries and freshly squeezed lemon juice, plus a bowl of hot millet cereal topped with sliced almonds	Small bowl of sugar snap peas	Falafel, tabbouleh and tahini in a pita (use falafel mix and premade, store-bought products)	Crisp-bread crackers spread with peanut butter and topped with sliced strawberries	Store-bought black bean burger topped with salsa and served with Oven-Baked Sweet Potato Fries (page 101)	Chilled watermelon and fresh mint drizzled with lime juice
Friday	Cashew "cream" with bananas (soak cashews overnight and then pulse in blender)	Medjool dates stuffed with almonds, served with a glass of soy milk	Store-bought vegan miso soup and Southeast Asian Summer Rolls with Peanut Dipping Sauce (page 104)	Raw zucchini slices with sundried tomatoes and store-bought vegan pesto	Red bell peppers stuffed with bulgur wheat, scallions, black beans and melted vegan cheese	Coconut Oatmeal Rum Raisin Cookies (page 108)

Week 2

	Breakfast	Snack	Lunch	Snack	Dinner	Snack
Saturday	Multigrain toast with nut butter and a bowl of blueberries	Kale chips	Steamed edamame, water chestnut and mushroom salad dressed with bottled soy-ginger marinade	Rhubarb applesauce with walnuts (just add cooked rhubarb to applesauce)	Cauliflower and vegan cheese sprinkled with nutmeg and served with brown rice pilaf	Strawberry-Kiwi Fizz (page 99) served with pretzels and a scoop of coconut milk ice cream
Sunday	Waffles with strawberries, maple syrup and vegan butter	Coconut milk and banana "shake" (mix the two ingredients in a blender)	Baked sweet potato topped with maple syrup and a pinch of nutmeg	Raw green beans and store-bought vegan artichoke dip	Store-bought veggie burger with lettuce, onion and tomato on a portobello "bun," served with mashed cauliflower (made with vegan butter)	Frosted Chocolate Fudge Brownies (page 112)

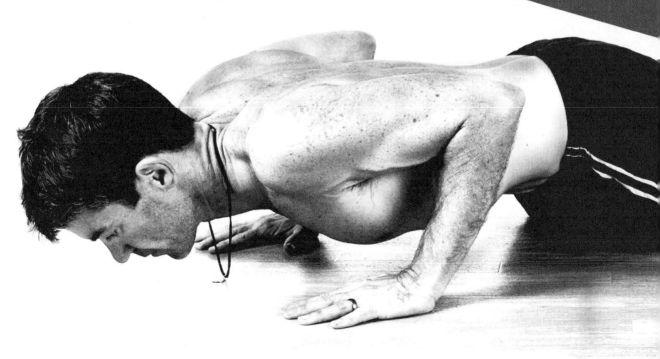

PART III:
FITNESS

VEGAN & FIT: THE EXERCISE PROGRAM

As personal trainers, we receive plenty of requests for an all-around fitness program to develop strength, speed, agility, endurance and full-body toning, but by far most clients are looking for a quick way to lose weight and get healthy. Luckily, the Vegan & Fit program can help you achieve all of those goals! Composed of easily repeatable bodyweight exercises and jogging intervals, this program is designed for athletes of all ages and abilities to progressively reach new fitness goals and develop a healthy, toned physique in as little as 20 minutes a day—without a gym membership or any complicated equipment.

Like this program and want even more? Vegan & Fit was adapted from *7 Weeks to Getting Ripped* and other fitness books by Brett Stewart. Learn more at www.7weekstofitness.com

Getting Started

This four-week program is a primer to rev up your metabolism and get you on track to getting—and staying—healthy and fit. Coupled with a clean vegan diet, the results of weight loss and reshaping your physique are entirely attainable!

Prior to beginning any physical fitness regimen, it's important to visit a physician and get medical clearance. A yearly check-up should be part of your maintenance plan to stay healthy and active.

Take this program at your own pace, especially if you're new to fitness or just getting active again after some time away. Use the program as a guideline for general fitness and skip moves that may be difficult while you're just getting the hang of it. There's no "four-week goal" associated with the program—the only goal is that you learn the exercises and develop your own sustainable routine to enjoy a lifetime of health and fitness. When you've completed the 12 workouts listed below, continue your progression by restarting the program and adding 1–3 repetitions to each exercise and 30 seconds to each of the timed planks.

What You'll Need

Vegan & Fit was designed to use your own body weight to strengthen, tone and develop agility, so you won't need any complicated equipment. A sturdy chair for dips, a solid-core door for door pull-ups, a digital timer or watch with a second hand for the timed exercises and an optional padded exercise mat are all the hardware you should require.

Dress in comfortable clothes that don't restrict your movement, grab a towel to wipe sweat from your hands and brow, and keep a bottle of water handy to hydrate between exercises.

Warming Up & Stretching

Properly warming up the body prior to any activity is very important, as is stretching post-workout. Please note that warming up and stretching are two completely different things: A warm-up routine should be done before stretching so that your muscles are more pliable and able to be stretched efficiently. You should not "warm up" by stretching; you simply don't want to push, pull or stretch cold muscles.

Prior to warming up, your muscles are significantly less flexible. Think of pulling a rubber band out of a freezer: If you stretch it forcefully before it has a chance to warm up, you'll likely tear it. Stretching cold muscles can cause a significantly higher rate of muscle strains and even injuries to joints that rely on those muscles for alignment.

It's crucial to raise your body temperature prior to beginning a workout. In order to prevent injury, such as a muscle strain, you want to loosen up your muscles and joints before you begin the actual exercise movement. A good warm-up before your workout should slowly raise your core body temperature, heart rate and breathing.

Before jumping into the workout, you must increase blood flow to all working areas of the body. This augmented blood flow will transport more oxygen and nutrients to the muscles being worked. The warm-up will also increase the range of motion of your joints.

A warm-up should consist of light physical activity (such as walking, jogging, stationary biking, jumping jacks, etc.) and only take 5–10 minutes to complete. Your individual fitness level and the activity determine how hard and how long you should go but, generally speaking, the average person should build up to a light sweat during warm-ups. You want to prepare your body for activity, not fatigue it.

The Program

Warm up for at least 5 minutes prior to beginning each daily exercise. To fire up your metabolism, each exercise is performed back to back with little or no time in between. If you feel fatigued, light-headed or dizzy, stop exercising and relax. If symptoms persist for more than a few minutes or intensify, seek medical help.

The repetitions listed are a guideline; if you can't complete all of the listed number of exercises per set, continue performing as many good-form exercises as you can. Add repetitions or sets to make the program more difficult if needed and cut down rest periods between sets.

You choose your own intensity. Executing each movement with proper form and adding explosive plyometric movements will help boost your fat burn and create a more demanding workout.

The program is based on three workout days a week, approximately 20 minutes in duration. Every other day is a rest day; on weekends try to spend at least 1 hour participating in a fitness activity.

Week 1

Sunday	1 hour fitness activity	**Thursday**	Rest day
Monday	**SET 1** 10 Push-Ups (Knee, Wall or Standard) (pages 62–64) 12 Squats (page 67) 10 Hip Raises (page 66) Rest 2:00 **SET 2** 12 Forward Lunges (6 each leg) (page 69) 10 Supermans (page 73) 8 Chair Dips (page 65) Rest 2:00 *Repeat Sets 1 & 2*	**Friday**	**SET 1** 12 Mountain Climbers (page 70) 3 Door Pull-Ups (page 75) 10 Hip Raises (page 66) Rest 2:00 **SET 2** 15 Reverse Crunches (page 72) 10 Supermans (page 73) :45 Plank (page 71) Rest 2:00 *Repeat Sets 1 & 2*
Tuesday	Rest day	**Saturday**	1 hour fitness activity
Wednesday	20/20 Drill (page 79)–Medium Intensity Rest 2:00 20/20 Drill (page 79)– High Intensity		

Week 2

Sunday	1 hour fitness activity		**Thursday**	Rest day
Monday	Run Intervals (page 88)		**Friday**	Stair Climbers (page 86)
Tuesday	Rest day		**Saturday**	1 hour fitness activity

Wednesday

SET 1

5 Inchworms (page 78)

10 Push-Ups (Knee, Wall or Standard) (pages 62–64)

6 Air Squats (page 68)

Rest 2:00

SET 2

12 Mountain Climbers (page 70)

3 Door Pull-Ups (page 75)

10 Hip Raises (page 66)

Rest 2:00

Repeat Sets 1 & 2

Week 3

Sunday	1 hour fitness activity	**Thursday**	Rest day

Monday

SET 1

10 Burpees (page 76)

10 Supermans (page 73)

:45 Plank (page 71)

Rest 2:00

SET 2

10 Push-Ups (page 64)

4 Door Pull-Ups (page 75)

16 Reverse Crunches (page 72)

Rest 2:00

Repeat Sets 1 & 2

Friday

SET 1

14 Bicycle Crunches (page 74)

6 Inchworms (page 78)

12 Chair Dips (page 65)

Rest 2:00

SET 2

8 Air Squats (page 68)

12 Mountain Climbers (page 70)

12 Hip Raises (page 66)

Rest 2:00

Repeat Sets 1 & 2

Tuesday

Rest day

Saturday

1 hour fitness activity

Wednesday

20/20 Drill (page 79)–Medium Intensity

Rest 2:00

20/20 Drill (page 79)–High Intensity

Week 4

Sunday	1 hour fitness activity		**Thursday**	Rest day
Monday	Stair Climbers (page 86)		**Friday**	Run Intervals (page 88)
Tuesday	Rest day		**Saturday**	1 hour fitness activity

Wednesday

SET 1

12 Burpees (page 76)

10 Supermans (page 73)

:45 Plank (page 71)

Rest 2:00

SET 2

12 Mountain Climbers (page 70)

3 Door Pull-Ups (page 75)

10 Hip Raises (page 66)

Rest 2:00

Repeat Sets 1 & 2

THE EXERCISES

Knee Push-Up

Knee push-ups are performed exactly as "standard" push-ups (page 64), but instead of your toes touching the ground, your knees will be the point of contact. This eliminates some of the weight of your legs and the smaller angle makes the movement about 15–25 percent easier.

1 Kneel and place your hands on the ground approximately shoulder-width apart. Walk your hands forward until your body forms a straight line from head to knees.

2 Inhale and lower your upper body toward the floor, stopping when your chest is about 3 inches from the floor.

Using your arms, chest, back and core, exhale and push your body back to starting position.

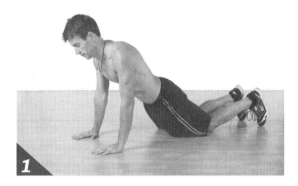

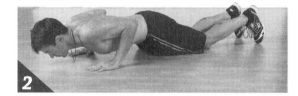

Wall Push-Up

This is easier than all floor push-ups, including those done from the knees.

1 Place your hands on a wall about shoulder-width apart and position your feet as far away from the wall as you feel comfortable. The farther your feet are from the wall, the harder the move will become. Engage your core to keep your back straight and your body in a straight line from head to feet; don't lean your head forward.

2 Inhale as you lower your entire body toward the wall, stopping before your head touches.

Exhale and, using your chest and arms, push your body away from the wall back to starting position.

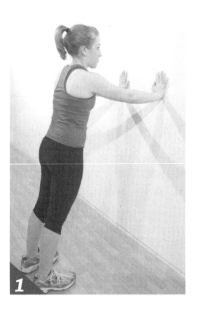 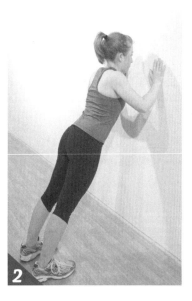

Push-Up

1 Place your hands on the ground approximately shoulder-width apart, making sure your fingers point straight ahead and your arms are straight but your elbows not locked. Step your feet back until your body forms a straight line from head to feet. Your feet should be about 6 inches apart with the weight in the balls of your feet. Engage your core to keep your spine from sagging; don't sink into your shoulders.

2 Inhale as you lower your torso to the ground and focus on keeping your elbows as close to your sides as possible, stopping when your elbows are at a 90-degree angle or your chest is 1–2 inches from the floor.

Using your shoulders, chest and triceps, exhale and push your torso back up to starting position.

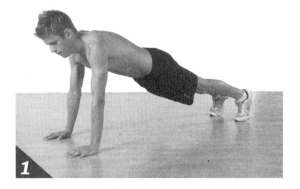

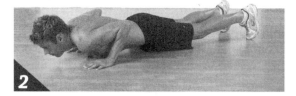

Chair Dip

A great way to build triceps and chest strength, dips are pretty convenient to do just about anywhere.

1 Sit on the very edge of a stable chair, place your palms next to your hips and grip the edge of the bench. Raise your butt off the bench and walk your feet out in front of you. Keep your legs straight and bend a little at your waist.

2 Inhale, bend your elbows and slowly lower your butt down toward the floor, stopping when your upper arms are at a 90-degree angle in relation to your lower arms.

Exhale and extend your arms until they're straight.

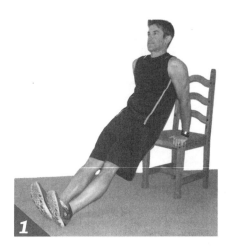
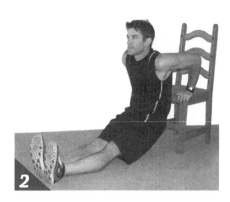

Hip Raise

This exercise is a slow and controlled motion that works the entire core—back, hips and abs—and provides a great way to work those muscles without any impact.

1 Lie on your back with your knees bent to about 90 degrees and feet flat on the floor. Extend your hands toward your hips and place your arms and palms flat on the floor at your sides.

2 Engage your abdominal muscles to keep your core tight, and exhale while you press your feet into the floor and raise your hips and lower back up, forming a straight line from your sternum to your knees. Do not push your hips too high or arch your back. Hold this position for 15–30 seconds. Inhale and slowly return to starting position.

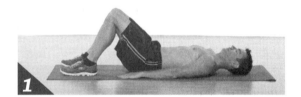 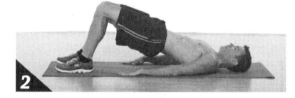

Squat

Squat form is crucial to getting the most out of this extremely beneficial exercise. Check out your form by standing perpendicular to a full-body mirror as you complete your reps.

1 Stand tall with your feet shoulder-width apart and toes pointed slightly outward, about 11 and 1 o'clock. Raise your arms until they're parallel to the floor.

2 Bend at the hips and knees and "sit back" just a little bit as if you were about to sit directly down into a chair. Keep your head up, eyes forward and arms out in front of you for balance. As you descend, contract your glutes while your body leans forward slightly so that your shoulders are almost in line with your knees. Your knees should not extend past your toes and your weight should remain between the heel and the middle of your feet—do not roll up on the balls of your feet. Stop when your knees are at 90 degrees and your thighs are parallel to the floor. If you feel your weight is on your toes or heels, adjust your posture and balance until your weight is in the middle of your feet. Squats should be a very stable movement—that is, until you try the one-legged variety!

Push straight up from your heels back to starting position. Don't lock your knees at the top of the exercise.

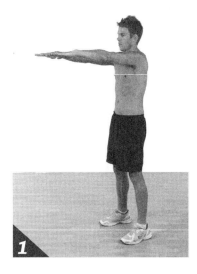
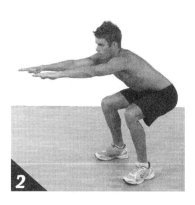

Air Squat

Adding an explosive jump to the top of your squat turns this already excellent full-body movement into a plyometric exercise to build even more strength, stamina and endurance.

1 Stand tall with your feet shoulder-width apart and toes pointed slightly outward, about 11 and 1 o'clock. Raise your arms until they're parallel to the floor. Bend at the hips and knees and "sit back" just a little bit as if you were about to sit directly down into a chair. Keep your head up, eyes forward and arms out in front of you for balance. As you descend, contract your glutes while your body leans forward slightly so that your shoulders are almost in line with your knees. Your knees should not extend past your toes and your weight should remain between the heel and the middle of your feet—do not roll up on the balls of your feet. Stop when your knees are at 90 degrees and your thighs are parallel to the floor.

2 Swing your extended arms down on both sides of your body until your hands are behind you. Pushing straight up from your midfoot, forcefully jump straight up in the air while swinging your arms forward and then straight overhead, pointing your fingers directly toward the ceiling.

Land softly on your forefeet with knees bent slightly to absorb the impact.

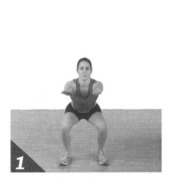

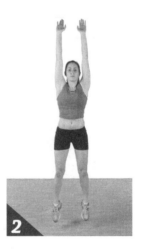

Forward Lunge

1 Stand tall with your feet shoulder-width apart and your arms hanging at your sides.

2 Take a large step forward with your right foot, bend both knees and drop your hips straight down until both knees are bent 90 degrees. Your left knee should almost be touching the ground and your left toes are on the ground behind you. Keep your core engaged and your back, neck and hips straight at all times during this movement.

Pushing up with your right leg, straighten both knees and return to starting position. Repeat with the other leg.

Reverse Variation: Reverse Lunges are just like their forward counterparts, but begin by taking a step backward. These can be slightly more difficult to maintain your balance and are a bit better for activating supporting muscles in your pelvis, legs and core.

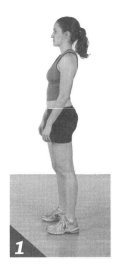
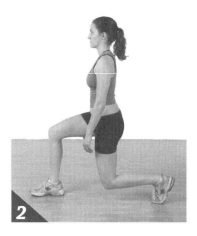

Mountain Climbers

1 Assume the top position of a push-up with your hands directly under your shoulders and toes on the ground. Keep your core engaged and your body in a straight line from head to toe.

2 Lift your right toe slightly off the ground, bring your right knee to your chest and place your right foot on the ground under your body.

3 With a very small hop from both toes, extend your right foot back to starting position and at the same time bring your left knee to your chest and place your left foot on the ground under your body.

Continue switching, making sure to keep your hips low.

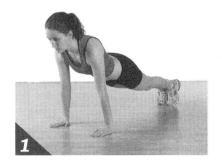
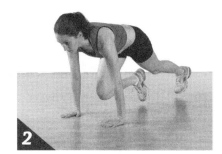
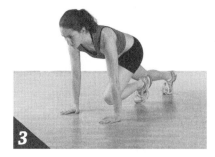

Plank

This is a timed exercise, so place a watch where you can see it when you're in position.

1 Place your hands on the ground approximately shoulder-width apart, making sure your fingers point straight ahead and your arms are straight but your elbows not locked. Step your feet back until your body forms a straight line from head to feet. Your feet should be about 6 inches apart with the weight in the balls of your feet. Engage your core to keep your spine from sagging; don't sink into your shoulders. Look at your watch and note the time—you're on the clock. Lower to starting position when time is reached.

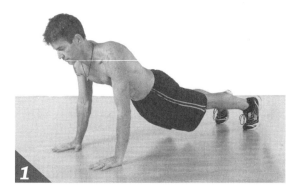

Forearm Variation: Place your elbows on the floor beneath your shoulders, your hands palm-down on the floor and your entire forearms in contact with the floor. Because your body is closer to parallel with the floor, you're working your core even harder to maintain a straight line from head to toe.

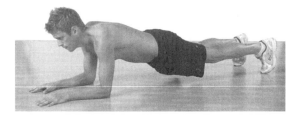

Reverse Crunch

Keep your back straight and lower legs on a level plane throughout this slow and controlled movement.

1 Lie flat on your back with your legs extended along the floor and your arms along your sides, palms down.

2 Contracting your lower abdominal muscles, lift your feet 4–6 inches off the floor, bend your knees and bring them in toward your chest. Be careful not to put excessive pressure on your lower back by bringing your hips off the floor. Pause when your glutes rise slightly off the mat.

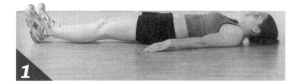

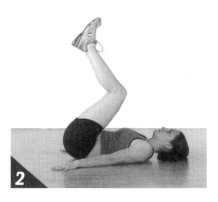

Superman

Interestingly enough, this exercise is not performed "up, up and away" but actually on your stomach, flat on the ground. However, the Man of Steel would greatly appreciate the importance of this move, as it strengthens your lower back and gives some due attention to your erector spinae—you know, those muscles that keep you vertical.

1 Lying face down on your stomach, extend your arms directly out in front of you and your legs behind you. Keep your knees straight as if you were flying.

2 In a slow and controlled manner, contract your erector spinae and raise your arms and legs about 6–8 inches off the floor. Hold for 5 seconds.

Lower slowly back to starting position.

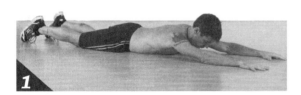
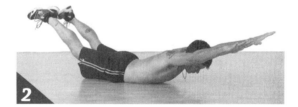

Bicycle Crunch

1 Lie flat on your back with your legs extended straight along the floor and your hands at both sides of your head, fingers touching your temples.

2 Raise your feet 6 inches off the floor while simultaneously contracting your rectus abdominis and lifting your upper back and shoulders off the floor. In one movement, bend your left knee and raise your left leg so that the thigh and shin are at 90 degrees; rotate your torso using your oblique muscles so that your right elbow touches the inside of your left knee.

3 Rotate your torso back to center and lower your upper body toward the floor, stopping before your shoulders touch.

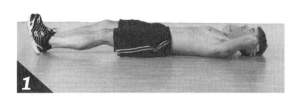

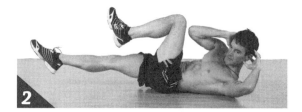

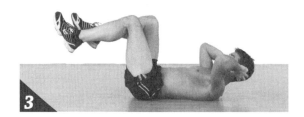

Door Pull-Up

These are a great way to get some training almost anywhere. The first step is to find a door that's sturdy enough to hold at least double your weight; you'll be putting a lot of stress on it. Solid-core doors with strong hinges are a must; hollow-core doors can crack and crumble. Also make sure that the top edge isn't sharp or slippery. Open the door in such a way to give yourself ample space to perform the exercise, and wedge a doorstop under it to keep it in place. The last thing you want to do is have the door close on your fingers!

1 Standing directly in front of the door, reach up and place your hands on top of it with your forearms flat on the front of it.

2 Using your forearms on the door as a lever, breathe out and engage the large muscles of your upper back and arms, bend your elbows and pull your chest up to the top of the door. If you need a little boost, jump up slightly at the start of the move.

Inhale as you slowly lower your feet back to the ground.

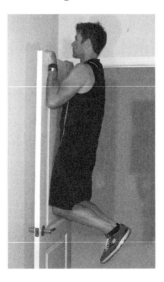

Burpee

The Burpee combines a squat, a double-leg mountain climber, a push-up and a high jump. It's a great full-body workout that you can do anywhere to work up a sweat and target your arms, chest, glutes, quads, hamstrings, calves and core. Since it's a multiple-position movement, take the time to learn and practice proper position for each move before you try it at full speed.

1 Stand tall with your back erect, feet shoulder-width apart and toes rotated slightly outward.

2 Shift your hips backward and "sit back" for the squat, keeping your head up and bending your knees. Lean your weight forward and place your hands on the floor, inside, outside or in front of your feet—whichever is more comfortable and gives you a nice, stable base.

3 Kick your feet straight back so that you're now in a push-up starting position, forming a nice line from your head to your feet. Keep your core tight to maintain an erect spine.

4 Inhale as you lower your torso toward the floor for a push-up. Stop when your body is 1–2 inches from the floor.

5 Exhaling, straighten your arms and propel your entire upper body off the floor while simultaneously bending your knees and bringing them toward your chest in order to plant your feet underneath you. You should end up back in the bottom position of a squat. Take a quick breath.

6 Swing your arms straight overhead, exhale and push off from your feet to jump straight up in the air as high as possible. Land with your knees slightly bent to absorb the impact. That's 1 rep.

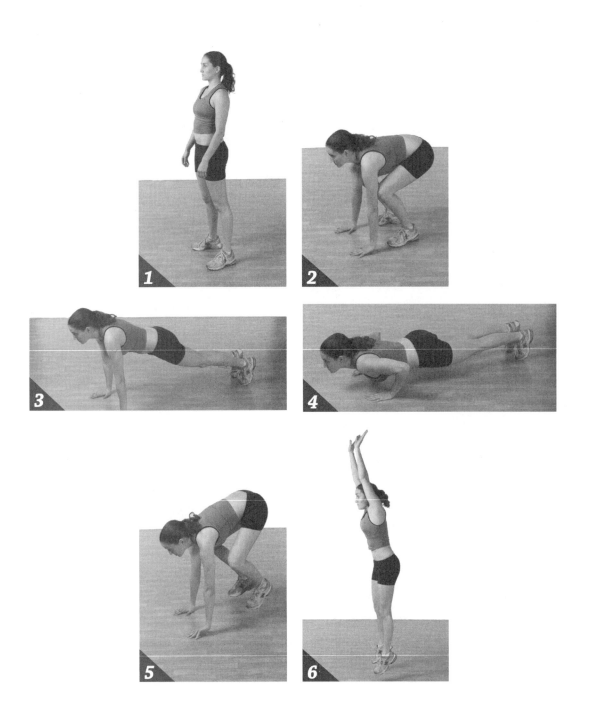

Inchworm

This is a great full-body exercise and a perfect test for hamstring and lower back flexibility. In this motion-based exercise, you'll advance forward approximately 4 feet per repetition, so plan your exercise positioning accordingly.

1 Stand with your feet about hip-width apart and fold over so that your hands touch the floor.

2–3 Keeping your hands firmly on the floor to balance your weight, walk your hands out in front of you one at a time until you're at the top of a push-up. Hold for 3 seconds.

4–5 Keeping your hands firmly on the floor to balance your weight, "walk" your feet toward your head by taking very small steps on your toes. Imagine that your lower legs are bound together and you can only bend your feet at each ankle. As you continue walking your feet toward your head, your butt will rise and your body will form an inverse "V." When you've stretched your hamstrings, glutes and calves as far as you can, hold that position for 3 seconds. That's 1 rep.

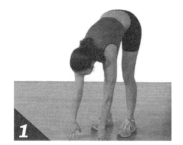
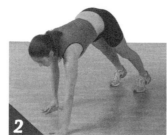
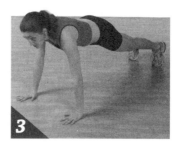

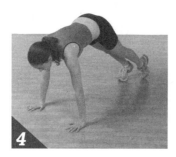
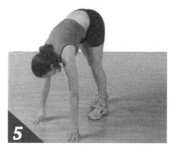

20/20 Drill

The 20/20 Drill combines eight different running-related mobility movements to develop speed, strength, flexibility and, most of all, endurance. The set-up is simple: Find a flat(ish) field at least 20 yards long and place some cones or markers at each end. You'll perform each of these movements back to back with little or no rest in between. Run 20 yards out, turn around and run 20 yards back—simple. The hard part is finding your rhythm and pushing yourself to keep the intensity up for each of these eight movements.

High Knees   Run forward using a normal-length stride. Bend the knee of your elevated leg 90 degrees and raise it until it's level with your waist. Push forward from the ball of your grounded foot, switch legs and repeat. Pump your arms to generate leg drive and speed.

When you've completed 20 yards of High Knees, turn around and perform Butt Kicks back to the starting position.

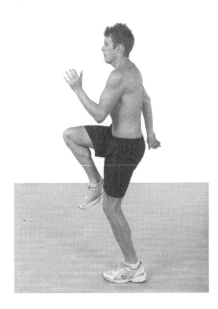

Butt Kicks   Run forward by taking very small steps and raising the heel of your back leg up toward your buttocks. Push forward from the ball of your grounded foot, progressing 12 to 18 inches per stride.

Turn around and perform 20 yards of Striders.

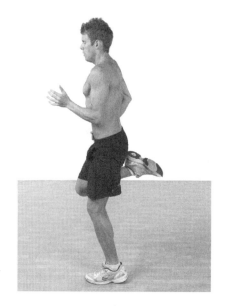

Striders   Bound forward by pushing off hard from the ball of your grounded foot, pumping your arms to generate leg drive and speed. Take huge leaps forward, trying to cover as much ground as possible with each stride.

After you've finished 20 yards of Striders, turn around and Skip back to the starting position.

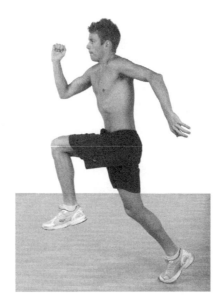

Skip   Bound forward by pushing off hard from the ball of your grounded foot, landing again on that same foot, and pushing off once more before landing on the opposite foot. Pump your arms to generate leg drive and speed. Take smaller leaps forward than when performing Striders, covering slightly less ground per stride.

Turn sideways and perform 20 yards of Side Shuffle.

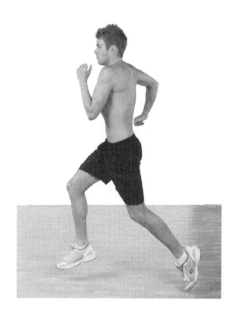

Side Shuffle   Turn sideways with your left hip pointing toward the direction you'll be traveling, feet slightly wider than your shoulders and hands at your side. Push off with your right foot in the direction you'll be traveling while lifting your left foot and swinging your right foot toward the center of your body. Touch both feet together lightly before landing on your right foot, extending your left foot out to the side in the direction you're traveling and repeating the process.

When you reach the 10-yard mark, turn 180 degrees so that your right hip is pointing in the direction that you're traveling and continue side shuffling an additional 10 yards.

Once you've completed 20 yards, turn to face the starting position and perform 20 yards of Walking Lunges.

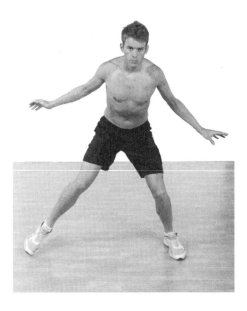

Walking Lunge   Stand tall, facing the direction you'll be traveling, with your feet shoulder-width apart and your arms hanging at your sides. Take a large step forward with your right foot, bend both knees and drop your hips straight down until both knees are bent 90 degrees. Your left knee should almost be touching the ground and your left toes are on the ground behind you. Keep your core engaged and your back, neck and hips straight at all times during this movement.

Keeping your right foot in place on the ground, push up with your right leg, straighten both knees and bring your legs to parallel, placing your left foot right next to your right.

Continue moving forward by repeating the above process with your left foot.

When you reach the start line, continue facing the same direction as you did during the Walking Lunge and perform Backward Sprints for 20 yards.

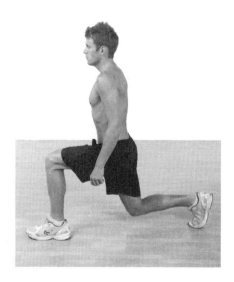

Backward Sprint   Facing away from the direction you'll be traveling, run by pushing off alternating forefeet and raising your knees as high as possible. Pump your arms as needed to generate leg drive and speed. This takes a little getting used to but it's a great way to strengthen your running muscles by working them in an opposite plane of motion and helps to develop balance and agility.

Once you've reached the 20-yard mark, lower your hand to the ground with both knees bent in a starter's stance and then Sprint as hard as you can back to the starting line.

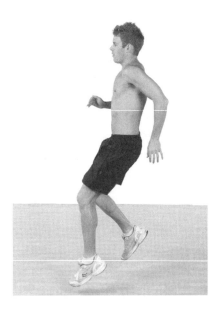

Sprint   The sprint is saved for last so you're working extremely hard to generate speed after your legs and lungs are already fatigued. Run forward at top speed by leaning forward with your upper body to as much as a 45-degree angle and driving off the balls of your feet as hard and as rapidly as you can. Pump your arms to increase leg drive and speed.

Stair Climbers

Find a set of stairs with 10–15 steps. Stair running is a great way to build up your quadriceps and calf strength as well as develop cardiovascular endurance.

Warm-Up   Run up one stair at a time, jog back down
5 FLIGHTS
REST :30

Quick Feet   Sprint up the flight of stairs as quickly as you can! Pump your arms to create leg turnover and practice "light feet" by making as little contact with the steps as possible.
3 FLIGHTS
REST :30

Doubles   Jump off one foot and bound up 2 steps at a time. Jog down 1 step at a time.
2 FLIGHTS
REST :30

Lunge-Ups   Starting at the bottom, raise your right foot and place it two steps up. Keeping your torso erect (see Forward Lunge on page 69), drop straight down until your right leg forms a 90-degree angle; your left knee should descend toward the first step. Be careful not to hit your knee on the edge of the step! Pressing through your right foot, raise your body back to a standing position and bring your left leg next to your right foot on the second step. That's 1 rep. Repeat up the rest of the staircase and then jog back down. This should be a slow, controlled exercise.
1 FLIGHT
REST :30

High Knee Steps Running up one step at a time, lift your knees as close to your chest as possible before placing your foot on the next step up. Jog back down.

3 FLIGHTS
REST :30

Hops Standing with both feet together, crouch down in a squat motion (see page 67) and, pushing from the balls of both feet, jump up as many stairs as you can and land squarely on the middle of the step with both feet, bending your knees to lessen the impact. Swinging your arms will help start your momentum and potentially increase your jump height. Jog down the stairs once you reach the top.

1 FLIGHT
REST 2:00

Repeat Quick Feet, Doubles, Lunge-Ups, High Knee Steps and Hops.

Run Intervals

These intervals will help you build up your mileage with two tempo runs of 1 mile each as well as 10 minutes of jogging to warm up and cool down. The hard sprints will help you develop speed and strength. When combined with the walking intervals, they'll help you develop endurance by progressively adding additional runs after slowing down and recovering.

Jog 5 minutes at an easy pace to warm up; rest for 1:00, hydrate and stretch your hips, calves and quads.

Run 1 mile at a moderate pace; rest for 1:00.

Run :40 at a hard pace, walk for :30.

Run :30 at a hard pace, walk for :30.

Run :20 at a hard pace, walk for :30.

Run :10 at a hard pace, rest for 1:00.

Run 1 mile at a moderate pace.

Jog 5 minutes at an easy pace to cool down.

Easy: You should be able to carry on a conversation and breathe relatively normally. An easy pace is good for warm-up, cool-down, recovery the day or two after a hard-run race, or when running long distances. Easy runs or jogs are roughly 50 percent of your maximal effort.

Moderate: Your breathing should be faster than normal due to your elevated heart rate and exertion. While you can't carry on a full conversation, you can speak in occasional sentences. Moderate, or tempo, runs help to build strength and endurance. Moderate runs are about 70 to 80 percent of your maximal effort.

Hard: This is all-out sprinting. You'll be breathing extremely hard and unable to speak more than a word or so at a time. Hard intervals are done for a short period of time to build speed and train fast-twitch muscle fibers to respond even when fatigued. Hard runs represent 95 percent of your maximal effort.

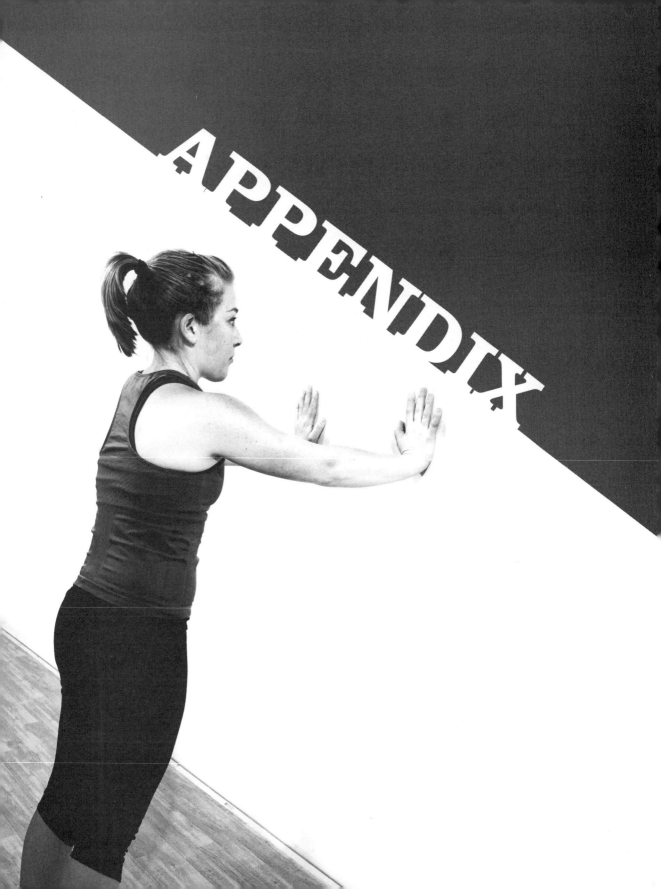

APPENDIX

COOKING VEGAN: THE RECIPES

The recipes in this book have been specifically tailored to the time-crunched athlete who doesn't have hours to mess around in the kitchen. The recipes are simple and straightforward, and incorporate everyday, readily available ingredients.

Note: Some of the following recipes contain honey. If you're a strict vegan and thus don't consume honey, you can modify the recipes by substituting molasses, maple syrup or applesauce in some instances.

Mushroom-Olive Quinoa Pilaf with Fresh Herbs

Quinoa is SO versatile and the perfect food for athletes. For starters, it's a complete protein, containing all nine amino acids, including large amounts of lysine, an amino acid essential to tissue growth and repair, helpful for post-exercise recovery. It's an excellent source of magnesium, iron, copper and phosphorus. It also contains a decent amount of tryptophan, so if you eat a large amount of it, make sure you've cleared your schedule for a three-hour nap. Quinoa is also supposed to be good for cardiovascular health and may help those with migraine headaches, asthma, atherosclerosis, breast cancer and/or diabetes. **4 SERVINGS AS A SIDE DISH, OR 2 SERVINGS AS A MAIN COURSE**

1 Tbsp. finely minced garlic (about 2 large cloves)

1 Tbsp. extra virgin olive oil

1 c. thinly sliced mushrooms (about 3 large mushrooms)

¼ tsp. salt

¼ tsp. ground black pepper

1 c. uncooked quinoa

¼ c. dry white wine

2½ c. water, plus more as needed

1 tsp. finely minced fresh rosemary leaves, densely packed

½ tsp. julienned fresh sage leaves, densely packed

½ c. Kalamata olives, pitted and sliced crosswise into ¼"-thick rounds (about 16 large olives)

¼ c. finely minced fresh Italian flat-leaf parsley, densely packed

¼ c. julienned fresh basil leaves, densely packed

½ c. shredded soy cheese

In a medium saucepan, sauté garlic in olive oil for 2–3 minutes on low heat. Do not let garlic brown. Next add mushrooms, season with salt and pepper, and gently stir to combine. Cook for another minute, then add quinoa. Stir ingredients until just combined, and cook for 1 minute more, allowing the quinoa to crisp slightly. Immediately add dry white wine to deglaze and cook until liquid has been reduced to a thin layer on the bottom of the pan, about 5 minutes. Pour in 2½ cups of water, stir to combine, cover with a lid and bring to a rolling boil. Reduce heat to low again and simmer for 10–15 minutes, or until water has been completely absorbed. With about 5 minutes of cooking time left to go, add fresh rosemary and sage, followed by the Kalamata olives.

During the final minute of cooking, lift the lid and taste for consistency; if the quinoa is still a bit too hard and crunchy, add more water as needed (i.e., a cup at a time, waiting until each cup has been absorbed before adding the next) and continue to cook until the grains soften a bit more to the desired consistency. Be careful not to overcook—you don't want it to be mushy; it should still have a slight crunch to it when it's done cooking, but it shouldn't be so hard that it'll break your teeth. When ready, remove from heat, remove the lid, add fresh parsley, basil and soy cheese, and stir until just combined. Cover once again and let stand for 10–15 minutes, then uncover and gently fluff once. Serve immediately.

Southwestern Black Bean Salsa Tortilla Wrap

This is a light and easy-to-make meal that's perfect for lunch. You can either eat one whole wrap that's been cut in half or only eat one half with a soup or salad. **6–8 WRAPS**

Black Bean Salsa Ingredients

1 (15.5 oz.) can black beans, drained and rinsed

½ c. diced yellow bell pepper (about ½ medium pepper)

¼ c. diced red onion (about ¼ small onion)

1½ Tbsp. finely diced seeded jalapeño (about ½ large jalapeño pepper)

1 c. diced fresh, vine-ripened tomatoes (about 3 small tomatoes)

1 c. shredded vegan Mexican four-cheese substitute blend

½ c. pitted, sliced ripe California olives (in ¼" rounds)

2 Tbsp. sliced scallions (green *and* white parts), in ¼" rounds (about 1 large scallion)

2 tsp. ground cumin

1 tsp. dried oregano leaves

pinch of salt (optional)

⅛ tsp. ground black pepper (or to taste)

⅛ tsp. ground chipotle pepper (or to taste)

2 Tbsp. finely minced fresh cilantro, densely packed

2 Tbsp. freshly squeezed lime juice (about 1 large lime)

1 c. diced Haas avocado (1 medium-sized Haas avocado)

Other Ingredients

4 c. *un*salted water (for cooking the corn)

½ c. frozen (or canned) corn kernels, thawed and drained

1 small romaine heart, leaves detached from base (½ large lettuce leaf, i.e., 4" piece, per person)

4–6 extra-large (i.e., 10" in diameter) low-fat flour tortillas

Make the salsa (in advance): In a large bowl, thoroughly mix all ingredients except for the avocado. Then add avocado and gently combine. (Avocado tends to get mushy quickly if mixed too vigorously.) Make sure all of the avocado is covered with lime juice, which will preserve it and keep it from oxidizing. Cover and place in the refrigerator until serving time. (It's better to let the ingredients marinate a bit; this produces a tastier end result.)

Next, steam the corn: Place a metal steamer basket into a large pot, and spread out its tabs so that it covers the entire bottom of the pot. Add roughly 4 cups of unsalted water to the pot, or however much water is needed to reach the base of the steamer. (Salted water toughens corn.) Bring water to a rolling boil over high heat, about 8 minutes. Add corn, cover pot with its lid, and steam for 2–3 minutes, or until tender. Drain into a colander. Allow to cool for a few minutes. Add steamed corn kernels to salsa and gently mix.

Assemble wraps: Place each tortilla onto a plate, then place half of a large romaine lettuce leaf (about a 4" piece) down the center of the tortilla. Next, place a line of black bean salsa down the center, about ¾ cup. (Don't overstuff tortillas with filling or the wrap will be hard to close.) Fold over the bottom end (i.e., the end that's closest to you) of the tortilla, bringing it up only about 2–3" toward the center. Then repeat for the opposite end. Starting from the sides of the tortilla that still remain open, roll the tortilla into a tight bundle. Slice wrap in half on the diagonal. Repeat with remaining ingredients. If you aren't serving them right away, wrap sandwiches in aluminum foil or waxed paper, and refrigerate until ready to serve.

Chef's Notes: You could also make the entire meal in advance and then take it to work for lunch. If you decide to do this, place salsa in a plastic container with a lid and the tortilla and lettuce leaf into separate resealable plastic bags. Tortillas tends to dry out and harden when exposed to air for too long.

As a variation on a theme, substitute baby spinach or mixed (i.e., mesclun) spring greens for the romaine lettuce. Spinach tastes very mild and thus doesn't distract from the flavor of the wrap, while mixed spring greens will add a bit of peppery flavor. For added flavor and color, you could also use spinach- or tomato-flavored low-fat flour tortillas. Colorful wraps make for a presentation that's pleasing to the eye as well as the stomach.

Chinese Eggplant and Tofu Stir-Fry

In this tasty Szechuan-style dish, the eggplants caramelize during the cooking process, and all of the flavors meld together into an ambrosial infusion of sweet and savory bliss. And the best part? All that deliciousness takes only minutes to prepare. **SERVES 2 AS A MAIN COURSE, OR 4 AS A SIDE DISH**

Sauce Ingredients

1 Tbsp. peanut butter

½ Tbsp. molasses

1 tsp. white rice wine vinegar

pinch of garlic powder

1 tsp. sesame seed oil

2 Tbsp. soy sauce

pinch of ground black pepper

Entrée Ingredients

2 Tbsp. sesame seed oil

2 Tbsp. finely minced fresh garlic (about 4 large cloves)

1 Tbsp. finely minced peeled fresh ginger (about 1" piece)

2 Tbsp. soy sauce

1 Tbsp. Chinese red rice wine vinegar (or, if unavailable, use white rice wine vinegar)

½ c. water

1 large (or 2 medium) Chinese eggplant, sliced lengthwise into ¼" x 3" strips (about 11–12 oz.) (if unavailable, use one 11–12 oz. regular eggplant)

1 Tbsp. tomato paste

¼ tsp. crushed red chili pepper flakes (or to taste)

1 c. diced firm tofu

¼ c. Thai sweet basil, tightly packed (if unavailable, use regular basil)

2 tsp. sesame seeds

In a small bowl, mix together stir-fry sauce ingredients until well combined and set aside. In a large wok, heat sesame oil on high heat for a few seconds until glistening, then reduce heat to low and sauté garlic and ginger for 2 minutes. Next, add soy sauce, red rice wine vinegar and water to deglaze, stirring on occasion, about 10–20 seconds. While liquid is reducing, add eggplant slices and cook until caramelized and light golden brown. Stir often so as not to let the eggplant burn or stick to the bottom of the pan. (Add more water as necessary.) After 3–4 minutes of cooking, stir in stir-fry sauce and tomato paste and then season with red chili pepper flakes, cooking until sauce mixture is thick and viscous. Next, add tofu and continue to cook. Add the basil during the last minute of cooking. Remove from heat and sprinkle with sesame seeds. If desired, serve atop a bed of jasmine rice with a side of steamed broccoli.

Chana Masala

Chana masala, also sometimes referred to as chole masala, is a savory, tangy chickpea and tomato dish commonly found on most (Northern) Indian and Pakistani restaurant menus. If you're going to serve the chana masala with rice, make the rice while the chana is cooking to save time. There are a zillion garam masala recipes out there, but this particular one was specifically created to complement this dish. To save time, consider making the garam masala in advance and storing it in an airtight container in a dark, dry place. **ABOUT 6 CUPS, OR 6–8 SERVINGS**

1 Tbsp. extra virgin coconut oil

2 c. diced Vidalia (or yellow) onion (about 1 medium onion)

2 Tbsp. julienned peeled fresh ginger, in 1" matchsticks

1 Tbsp. finely minced garlic

2 (15.5 oz.) can chickpeas (garbanzo beans)

1 (28 oz.) can crushed tomatoes

3 Tbsp. tomato paste

½ c. light coconut milk

2 Tbsp. garam masala (recipe follows)

½ Tbsp. amchur (dried mango powder), or to taste (if unavailable, substitute 1 Tbsp. freshly squeezed lemon juice, or to taste; see Chef's Note)

¼ tsp. ground turmeric

1½ c. diced fresh vine-ripened tomatoes (about 2½ small tomatoes)

¼ tsp. salt (or to taste)

½ c. fresh cilantro, roughly chopped

Garam Masala Ingredients

½ Tbsp. ground cumin

½ Tbsp. ground coriander

¾ tsp. ground cardamom

½ tsp. ground cinnamon

½ tsp. ground ginger

½ tsp. ground black pepper

⅛ tsp. ground clove

⅜ tsp. finely crushed bay leaves

¼ tsp. ground cayenne pepper (or to taste)

Heat extra virgin coconut oil in a large (12–13") sauté pan on medium heat until glistening. Reduce heat to low, add diced onions and ginger matchsticks and sauté until tender, about 3 minutes. Add garlic next and cook an additional 2 minutes. Next, add chickpeas, crushed tomatoes, tomato paste and coconut milk, and stir until well combined. Stir in garam masala, amchur and turmeric, and reduce liquid in pan by ¼ of its original volume. Be sure to stir continually so that sauce doesn't burn or stick to the bottom of the pan. Next, add vine-ripened tomatoes, season with salt and continue to cook just until tomatoes soften a bit. Be careful not to overcook tomatoes; they should still maintain their form and color and still have a slight crunch to them when you've finished cooking. (If the mixture cooks down too quickly, add water as necessary, ¼ cup at a time.) Remove from heat and divide into equal portions. Top with fresh chopped cilantro. Serve with jasmine rice and/or fresh, warm naan.

Chef's Note: If you'll be substituting lemon juice for the amchur, be sure to add it toward the end. Lemon juice's chemical composition becomes altered with heat, and will thus affect the other ingredients when it comes into contact with in the pan.

Penne with Cashew-Walnut Pesto and Sun-Dried Tomatoes

Pesto can be made in advance and refrigerated for up to four days or frozen for future use for about six to eight months. Store it in a tightly sealed container or plastic freezer bag. For easier and faster defrosting, place individual-sized portions in ice cube trays and then place trays into tightly sealed plastic freezer bags. Also, when you thaw pesto, you might need to add more lemon juice, as the flavor of the lemon juice tends to fade with freezing. **4 SERVINGS**

Pasta Ingredients

- 6 qts. lightly salted water, seasoned with a few drops of extra virgin olive oil
- 2 c. uncooked penne
- 1 c. julienned sun-dried tomatoes (buy precut kind to save time)
- ½ c. (or more) fresh basil leaves, densely packed, plus more for garnish
- 2 Tbsp. grated vegan Parmesan cheese

Pesto Ingredients (YIELD: ¾ CUP PESTO)

- 1 c. fresh basil leaves and stems, densely packed
- 2¼ tsp. minced garlic (about 1½ large cloves)
- ¼ c. lightly salted cashews
- ¼ c. chopped walnuts
- 3 Tbsp. extra virgin olive oil
- 1 Tbsp. freshly squeezed lemon juice
- ½ Tbsp. light silken tofu
- ⅛ tsp. salt

About a half hour before serving time, bring the water to a rolling boil in a medium stockpot. Add the penne and cook according to package instructions. While you're waiting for the water to boil, place all pesto ingredients in a food processor and pulse until well combined; set aside. When the pasta is ready, drain into a large colander, shock with cold running water, then drain again and pour back into the stockpot. Add pesto and sun-dried tomatoes and stir until pasta is well coated. Divide into equal portions and serve warm or at room temperature. Sprinkle each portion with vegan Parmesan cheese and small, julienned pieces of basil.

"Blueberry Blast" Breakfast Smoothie

2 (1-CUP) SERVINGS

1 c. frozen blueberries

½ c. crushed ice

½ c. plain (unsweetened) soy yogurt

1 Tbsp. honey

½ Tbsp. freshly squeezed lemon juice

Add all ingredients to a blender and pulse until smooth and frothy.

Watermelon-Coconut Sports Recovery Drink

This super-effective recovery drink has all the bases covered: It's rich in Omega-3s, zinc and powerful antioxidants that help reduce post-exercise inflammation, as well as essential electrolytes like potassium and magnesium, both of which are key to post-exercise recovery. It also contains the recommended 4:1 carbs-to-protein ratio to replenish glycogen stores and repair muscle. The fruits in this drink also naturally have a low glycemic load (GL), which not only stabilizes your blood sugar and increases your energy level, but is also helpful for losing pounds and maintaining your weight. Low-GL foods are slowly digested and metabolized, which provide a sustained source of energy for muscles.

For maximum effectiveness, be sure to consume this drink within the first 15–30 minutes after a workout. **3 CUPS**

¼ c. pitted medjool dates

½ c. diced seedless watermelon

2 Tbsp. red raspberries

2 Tbsp. freshly squeezed lime juice

½ c. coconut water

½ c. cold, brewed green tea (I use *Salada Green Tea with Purple Antioxidants*, which provides extra antioxidants and also naturally enhances the drink's reddish-pink color)

1 c. organic unsweetened soy milk

Place all solid ingredients into the blender and pulse until just combined. Then add liquids and pulse until smooth. Pour into a 1-gallon pitcher and cover with lid. Store in fridge and use throughout the week for post-exercise recovery.

Unbelievably Creamy and Delicious, "I-Can't-Believe-It's-Vegan," All Natural, Hot and Spicy, Sugar-Free Cocoa

This recipe is not only easy to make, but infinitely healthier and far less caloric than the traditional hot cocoa recipe. This is a truly yummy guilty pleasure but without the guilt, and who doesn't love that?! This cocoa actually has healing properties as well: Honey soothes the throat; cocoa powder stimulates the brain, wards off disease and stress, and elevates one's mood; cayenne pepper has anti-inflammatory properties, protects against colds and infections, and helps to clear one's respiratory passages; and coconut milk has many immunity-boosting properties. Coconut milk also just so happens to have built-in weight control attributes as well. **1 SERVING**

2 Tbsp. cocoa powder

⅛ tsp. ground cayenne pepper (or to taste; optional)

pinch of salt

2 Tbsp. honey (strict vegans can substitute 2 Tbsp. organic unsulphured blackstrap molasses)

½ c. water

1 c. light coconut milk

½ tsp. pure vanilla extract

Place cocoa powder, cayenne pepper, salt and honey in the bottom of a large mug and stir until the mixture turns into a thick, syrupy consistency. Set aside. Fill a tea kettle with water, put the kettle on, and then boil the water on high until the whistle blows. Measure ½ cup of boiling water in a metal measuring cup, then carefully pour it into the tea cup. Stir thoroughly until dissolved, wait about a minute or so, then add coconut milk and vanilla. Serve immediately (while piping hot!).

Strawberry-Kiwi Fizz

This drink will not only help you stay cool and hydrated, but it also smells as good as it tastes. It really hits the spot, especially on a sizzling summer's day. Instead of traditional cocktails at a summer party, serve a pitcher of strawberry-kiwi fizz and, if you like, spike it with a bit of vodka or gin. **78.8 FL. OZ., OR ABOUT 1 LARGE PITCHER**

2 Tbsp. finely minced mint

1 c. thinly sliced limes, in ¼" rounds (about 1½ large limes)

1 c. hulled and sliced strawberries

1 c. peeled and thinly sliced kiwis, in ¼" rounds

1 liter bottle seltzer water

½ c. honey (or to taste; substitute with the natural sweetener of your choice or omit altogether)

2 c. ice cubes

Add mint and limes to a glass pitcher. Mull these ingredients by pressing them against the sides of the pitcher with a spoon. Add all other ingredients, first solid ingredients followed by liquid ones, to pitcher and stir until well blended or until honey has dissolved. Add ice cubes just before serving. Serve immediately.

Chef's Note: Don't let this drink sit for too long or the mint in it will turn bitter.

Niña Colada Punch

This recipe is great for entertaining, and it's a real crowd-pleaser too! The basic recipe template is very versatile; substitute tofu for the ice cream to make a smoothie. Omit the ice cream to make a nonalcoholic cocktail. Or simply leave everything as is and add rum to make piña colada punch. **ABOUT 1 GALLON, OR 16 (1-CUP) SERVINGS**

2 c. unsweetened pineapple juice (not from concentrate!)

1 c. unsweetened pineapple juice, frozen into ice cubes

3 (13.5) fl. oz. cans light unsweetened coconut milk

¼ c. plus 1 Tbsp. honey

¼ c. lime juice

1 c. club soda

2 scoops coconut (or vanilla) soy or other nondairy ice cream

Add all ingredients except the ice cream into a blender in batches, and pulse until well blended and smooth. Add ice cream. Serve immediately.

Oven-Baked Sweet Potato Fries

Want to reduce post-exercise inflammation? Then eat these oven-baked sweet potato fries, which have very strong anti-inflammatory properties. With 23,017 mcg of beta-carotene per cup, sweet potatoes are a better source of beta-carotene than most leafy green vegetables. Even better, the small amount of fat in this recipe helps our absorption of that beta-carotene. Sweet potatoes are also high in vitamin A (38,433 IU), fulfilling 769% of the Recommended Daily Allowance (RDA). With all of their complex carbohydrates and excellent antioxidative proteins (sporamins), they're not only a high-satiety food but are also excellent for stabilizing blood sugar. With all of these benefits, plus their yummy, crunchy taste, what more reason do you need to take a bite? **2–4 SERVINGS**

1 lb. sweet potatoes, scrubbed and *unpeeled* (about 1 extra-large or 2 small sweet potatoes)

¼ c. extra virgin olive oil

1 Tbsp. cornstarch (to make fries crispy)

2 tsp. ground cumin

1 Tbsp. paprika

¼ tsp. kosher salt (or to taste)

¼ tsp. ground black pepper (or to taste)

⅛ tsp. ground cayenne pepper (or to taste)

½ tsp. garlic powder

½ tsp. onion powder

Preheat oven to 450°F and position a rack in the top of oven. Using a chef's knife, slice sweet potato into quarters, then again lengthwise into ¼"-thick slices, with the peel side facing up. Lay each slice flat and cut into long, ⅜"-thick strips. Put into a large shallow bowl and pour in olive oil, followed by the cornstarch and all of the spices. Toss together with your hands until sweet potatoes are thoroughly and evenly coated with oil and spices. Using tongs, shake off excess oil into the bowl and transfer sweet potatoes to two 11" x 17" baking trays covered with aluminum foil (for easy cleanup, or two disposable, 11" x 17" aluminum baking trays), placing potatoes in a single layer spaced evenly apart. Transfer both trays to the top shelf of the 450°F oven and bake for 22–25 minutes, or until golden brown. Allow to cool for a few minutes. Then use tongs to transfer to a large, paper-towel-covered tray to drain excess oil. (You can also pat them with another paper towel to blot more oil.) Divide into equal portions and serve immediately.

Aromatic Basmati Rice (Pilau)

This Indian-style recipe, also sometimes referred to as pilau ("fragrant rice") is aptly named. It's very simple and easy to make, and its wonderful aroma will fill your entire kitchen. For a complete meal, we suggest that you pair it with Chana Masala (page 95). **4 SERVINGS**

2 c. water

1 c. brown basmati rice

1 Tbsp. extra virgin olive oil

1 large bay leaf

3 (3") cinnamon sticks, broken in half

5 whole cloves

14 whole green cardamom pods

1 tsp. fennel seeds

1 tsp. cumin seeds

1 tsp. ground coriander

½ tsp. ground ginger

¼ tsp. ground turmeric

¼ tsp. onion powder

1½ tsp. saffron threads, soaked in 2 Tbsp. organic unsweetened plain soy milk and then stirred to combine

¼ tsp. salt (or to taste)

⅛ tsp. ground black pepper (or to taste)

1½ Tbsp. fresh cilantro (for garnish)

Stovetop Directions: Wash the rice by placing it into a large strainer, running it under cold water, and then swishing it around until the water runs clear. (This will remove any excess starch coating the rice.) Feel free to use your fingers to swirl the rice around in the strainer to ensure it is thoroughly washed. Drain and set aside over a small bowl. Heat olive oil in a medium saucepan on high heat until glistening. Add bay leaf, cinnamon sticks, cloves, cardamom pods, fennel seeds and cumin seeds and "flash fry" for 60 seconds to release the spices' essences, covering pan with a splatter screen to avoid being burned by sputtering oil. Reduce heat to low, add rice and cook for 1 minute more, stirring occasionally. Watch closely so the rice doesn't burn; rice will be a light golden brown when ready. (This is done to crisp the rice and keep it from getting soggy as it cooks while immersed in water.) Reduce heat to low, add water and coriander, ginger, turmeric, onion powder and saffron mixture and stir. For al dente rice, cover with a tight-fitting lid and simmer for 15 minutes or until water has been completely absorbed. (Check on rice after 15 minutes to make sure it hasn't cooked down too quickly. If it needs to cook for longer, add water as necessary.) Remove from heat and let rice rest for about 10 minutes. With a spoon, remove bay leaf, cinnamon sticks, cloves and cardamom pods and discard. Fluff rice with a fork, then sprinkle cilantro into the pot, stirring just until combined. Divide into 4 portions and serve immediately.

Rice Steamer Directions: Wash the rice by placing it into a large strainer, running it under cold water, and then swishing it around until the water runs clear. (This will remove any excess starch coating the rice.) Feel free to use your fingers to swirl the rice around in the strainer to ensure it is thoroughly washed. Drain and set aside over a small bowl. Add olive oil to rice steamer, followed by rice, water and all spices except for the cilantro, in the order listed. Stir once to combine and cover with inner steamer tray and lid. For al dente rice, cover with a tight-fitting lid and simmer for 15 minutes or until water has been completely absorbed. (Check on rice after 15 minutes to make sure it hasn't cooked down too quickly and/or burned on the bottom. If it needs to cook for longer, add water as necessary.) If steamer doesn't have a timer with an auto shut-off feature, turn it off when rice has finished cooking. Let rice rest for about 10 minutes. With a spoon, remove bay leaf, cinnamon sticks, cloves and cardamom pods and discard. Fluff rice with a fork, then sprinkle cilantro into the steamer, stirring just until combined. Divide into 4 portions and serve immediately.

Chef's Note: A rice steamer will cook rice more quickly than the stovetop method, plus it's a lot easier this way. Many, if not most, rice steamers have a built-in timer with an auto shut-off feature; there's usually a button you can depress to cook the rice, and it releases with a pop when the rice is done. Typically, this will take about 15–20 minutes, although you can cook it for longer if you like your rice a bit softer.

Southeast Asian Summer Rolls with Peanut Dipping Sauce

Unlike spring rolls, summer rolls are served raw and cold. They're popular throughout Southeast Asia (e.g., Vietnam, Thailand, Laos). In Asian restaurants, they're sometimes listed on the menu as "garden rolls," "fresh spring rolls," "fresh rolls" or sometimes "summer garden rolls." Even though the traditional version isn't vegan, of course this particular recipe is. **10 ROLLS, OR 5 SERVINGS OF 2 ROLLS PER PERSON**

Peanut Dipping Sauce Ingredients

1 c. dry-roasted unsalted peanuts

1 Tbsp. minced garlic (about 4 medium cloves)

1 Tbsp. minced peeled fresh ginger (about 1" piece)

¼ tsp. salt

⅛ tsp. crushed red chili pepper flakes

2 Tbsp. finely minced fresh cilantro, densely packed

3 Tbsp. freshly squeezed lime juice

2 Tbsp. soy sauce

2 Tbsp. honey (or substitute with molasses)

2 Tbsp. sesame seed oil

½ c. light unsweetened coconut milk (from a can)

¼ c. water (or more if necessary)

1 Tbsp. sesame seeds

Summer Roll Ingredients

1 c. cubed firm tofu, in ½" cubes

¼ c. julienned carrots, in 1½" matchsticks

½ c. shredded cabbage or lettuce

¼ c. mung bean sprouts

½ c. julienned cucumber, in 1½" matchsticks

½ c. julienned scallions (green and white parts), in 1½"-long matchsticks

¼ c. julienned mushrooms

2 Tbsp. finely minced fresh cilantro leaves, densely packed

2 Tbsp. finely minced mint leaves, densely packed

2 Tbsp. finely minced sweet Thai basil (use regular, if unavailable), densely packed

2 Tbsp. freshly squeezed lime juice

1 (3½" x 3½") brick vermicelli rice ("cellophane") noodles (makes about 1 c. cooked)

10 sheets vermicelli rice paper wrappers

1 c. sliced Haas avocado (about 1 avocado)

Make the peanut dipping sauce: (This step can be done in advance to reduce meal-time prep. Sauce will keep in the fridge for several days.) Add all sauce ingredients, minus the sesame seeds, into a food processor, pulse until smooth and transfer ingredients to a small saucepan. Cook for 3–4 minutes on medium-low heat, or until raw garlic smell disappears, stirring continually to avoid browning it on the bottom. (Add more water as necessary to prevent burning and achieve desired consistency.) Set aside. Gently fold in sesame seeds until combined.

Assemble the summer rolls: Place all summer roll ingredients (minus the vermicelli rice noodles, vermicelli rice paper and avocado) into a large bowl and toss until well combined. Chill in the refrigerator until serving time. About 15–20 minutes before serving time, bring a medium pot of water to a rolling boil, about 8 minutes, and add vermicelli noodles; boil for another 4 minutes. Remove pot from stove, drain noodles into a colander, rinse with cold water, and then drain again. Allow to cool completely. When ready to serve, place 1 sheet of vermicelli rice paper in a large bowl filled with hot water for about 10 seconds until completely moistened. Remove it from the water and lay it across a large plate. Place a ½ cup of the vegetable mixture onto the rice paper wrap, then lay an avocado slice on top. Gently lift up two opposite ends of the rice paper wrapper and fold them inward toward the center of the wrapper. Next, gently lift up an open, adjacent side of the wrapper and tuck it over the filling; roll the wrapper forward until the final, remaining end has been sealed. (Use a slight amount of pressure when tucking and rolling so that the roll is somewhat tightly wrapped, but don't pull or stretch too vigorously or the wrapper paper will tear. It's pliable and can take a bit of expansion, but it's not Silly Putty.) Repeat with remaining ingredients. Serve with peanut dipping sauce. Serve immediately (or at least within an hour of making them) for the best flavor and consistency.

Chef's Note: IMPORTANT—When shopping for the vermicelli rice paper, make sure you buy the ones labeled "fresh spring roll rice paper," sometimes marked as *bánh tráng gỏi cuốn* in Vietnamese. The other kinds require cooking.

The trick to easily handling the rice paper is not to leave it soaking in the hot water for too long; otherwise it'll become way too soft, and then will weaken and very likely tear. Also, it helps if you lay the rice paper on a plate that's slightly wet on the bottom, which prevents it from sticking to the plate. Once you soak the wrapper in the hot water to soften it, it's important to work quickly so that the paper sticks together and seals after you roll it.

Cucumber, Tomato and Artichoke Salad

Here's an easy salad recipe to make for lunch or dinner. The dressing is made with fresh herbs, which brings out the flavors of the salad ingredients. **MAKES 5 CUPS**

Salad Ingredients

1 medium cucumber, unpeeled

1 c. halved grape tomatoes (about 14 tomatoes)

1 (14 oz.) can plain artichoke hearts, drained and rinsed (about 1½ c.)

¼ c. finely minced fresh Italian flat-leaf parsley, densely packed

¼ c. julienned basil

Lemon Vinaigrette Salad Dressing

¼ c. freshly squeezed lemon juice

¼ c. extra virgin olive oil

¼ tsp. Dijon mustard

2 tsp. finely minced garlic (about 2 medium cloves)

1 Tbsp. fresh thyme leaves, densely packed

½ Tbsp. roughly chopped fresh marjoram leaves, densely packed

⅛ tsp. crushed red chili pepper flakes

⅛ tsp. ground black pepper

⅛ tsp. salt

Score the cucumber vertically all the way around with the tines of a fork, then dice and measure about 2 cups. Combine diced cucumber and remaining salad ingredients in a bowl and set aside. Combine salad dressing ingredients in a jar, seal tightly and shake to combine. Pour dressing over salad and toss. Let marinate (in the fridge in a covered container) for at least a half hour before serving to allow the flavors to meld.

Mexican-Style Gazpacho

Rich in antioxidants, electrolytes and Omega-3 fatty acids, this soup is a superfood extravaganza! The ingredients in this soup promote cardiovascular and eye health, regulate blood sugar levels, increase nutrient absorption, lower cholesterol levels, help fight cancer and provide a wide range of anti-inflammatory benefits, which are of course useful in reducing post-exercise soreness, among other things. Drink this soup and you'll be drinking to your health! **3–4 SERVINGS**

3 c. grape tomatoes

1 c. diced cucumber, half peeled (see Chef's Note)

½ c. diced red onion (about ¼ small onion)

2 Tbsp. minced garlic (about 4 large cloves)

½ c. diced Haas avocado (½ avocado)

¼ c. fresh mint leaves, densely packed

2 Tbsp. fresh cilantro, densely packed

1 tsp. dried oregano

1 tsp. ground cumin

½ tsp. kosher salt (or to taste)

¼ tsp. ground black pepper (or to taste)

⅛ tsp. Tabasco sauce (or to taste)

¼ c. red wine vinegar

¼ c. freshly squeezed lime juice

3 c. V-8 tomato juice (for milder gazpacho, add another ½ c.)

Optional Garnishes

3–4 Tbsp. shredded vegan cheese (about 1 Tbsp. per serving)

½ c. sliced Haas avocado (½ avocado)

fresh mint and/or cilantro leaves, finely minced

¼ c. sliced scallion (green and white parts), in ¼"-thick rounds

Add all solid ingredients to a blender, pulse to combine, then add liquids and pulse again until desired consistency has been reached. Divide into equal portions and pour into bowls. Top each portion with avocado slices, shredded soy cheese and/or other desired garnishes. Serve chilled or at room temperature.

Chef's Note: For higher nutritional value, peel the cucumber in alternating vertical stripes. This way, you'll preserve more of the nutrient-rich peel.

Coconut Oatmeal Rum Raisin Cookies

Moist, chewy and crisp around the edges, these are loaded with healthy, delicious ingredients. Coconut is excellent for athletes because it provides an immediately usable but sustainable source of energy. Coconut oil contains lauric acid, a medium-chain triglyceride (MCT) that actually helps the body to rapidly burn fat. Since the body can't readily store MCTs, it must burn them, thus resulting in an increase in fat oxidation and energy expenditure. Ingesting coconut oil in moderation can thus lead to weight loss.

Raisins are one of the best sources of boron, a mineral that's essential to bone health, and have been shown to provide protection against osteoporosis. Oats are a decent source of fiber, protein and carbohydrates, and have very strong anti-inflammatory properties. Oats also stabilize blood sugar, lower cholesterol, protect the heart, boost the immune system and lower the risk of type-2 diabetes.

Lastly, organic, unsulphured blackstrap molasses, which is what gives these cookies their distinct dark brown color and rich flavor, is actually good for you, unlike refined sugar. It contains a variety of minerals: iron, calcium, copper, magnesium, manganese, potassium, selenium and vitamin B6. **MAKES ABOUT 3 DOZEN COOKIES**

¼ c. ground golden flaxseeds

¾ c. water

2 c. extra virgin coconut oil

1 c. organic, unsulphured blackstrap molasses

3 tsp. pure vanilla extract

½ c. rum

2 c. coconut flour

1 tsp. salt

3 tsp. baking powder

3 tsp. baking soda

1¼ tsp. ground nutmeg

1¼ tsp. ground clove

¼ c. ground cinnamon

3 c. oats

½ c. unsweetened shredded coconut

2 c. dark seedless raisins

Preheat oven to 350°F. Pour ground flaxseeds into a small bowl, add water and stir until well combined. Allow mixture to sit for about 10 minutes, or until it puffs up a bit and forms a gel. (This mixture replaces eggs as the binding agent for the cookie dough.) Set aside. In a large bowl, mix together coconut oil, molasses, vanilla, rum, and flaxseed mixture until well-combined and smooth; set aside. Next, mix together all dry ingredients—minus the oats, shredded coconut and raisins—and then gradually incorporate the dry into the wet ingredients and mix well, until combined. By hand, fold in oats, coconut and raisins until well combined. Drop about ¼ cup of cookie dough onto an ungreased, parchment-covered cookie sheet. Flatten dough slightly using a fork. Repeat with remaining dough. Bake at 350°F for 12 minutes, or until light golden brown. Cool completely on wire rack. Store in an airtight container to keep cookies soft and chewy.

Pear and Apple Crisp

This is a much healthier, vegan version of a popular favorite. Both pears and apples contain the flavenoid quercetin, which supports bone health and bolsters the immune system, among other benefits. Both fruits also have anti-inflammatory and antioxidative properties. So this probably explins why "an apple a day keeps the doctor away." **6–8 SERVINGS**

Filling Ingredients

1½ Tbsp. ground cinnamon

1 tsp. grated orange zest

½ tsp. grated lemon zest

⅛ tsp. salt

¼ tsp. ground nutmeg

¼ tsp. ground clove

¼ tsp. ground allspice

1 tsp. pure vanilla extract

2 Tbsp. orange juice

2 Tbsp. freshly squeezed lemon juice

2½ c. peeled, sliced ripe Bosc pears, in 1½" pieces (about 2½–3 large pears)

2½ c. peeled, sliced Granny Smith apples, in 1½" pieces (about 2 large apples)

Topping Ingredients

½ c. oats, finely ground in food processor into "oat flour"

¾ c. whole oats

⅛ tsp. salt

2 Tbsp. honey (or, for strict vegans, substitute applesauce)

2 Tbsp. organic unsweetened plain soy milk

1 Tbsp. cold vegan butter, cut into small cubes

Preheat oven to 350°F. Mix the cinnamon, orange zest, lemon zest, salt, nutmeg, clove and allspice in a small bowl. Stir in vanilla, orange juice and lemon juice. Set aside. Combine diced apples and pears in a large bowl, pour in the wet spice mixture and fold together until well combined. Transfer into a circular 1½-quart glass or stoneware baking dish that's about 8" across in diameter. (This size dish provides the perfect amount of surface area so that the topping will completely cover the filling.) Set aside. In the bowl of an electric mixer, combine the topping ingredients and mix on medium-low speed until mixture is well combined. When ready, mixture will form into small crumbly pieces. Using a spatula, scoop out the crumbly oat topping and place onto the filling's surface. Be sure to completely cover the filling with topping. Place baking dish onto a large baking tray (to keep your oven's interior clean if crisp should bubble over.) Place tray into oven and bake (uncovered) on 350°F for about 55–60 minutes or until crisp. Serve in little custard dishes with a scoop of vanilla soy ice cream.

Mango Pie with Cardamom and Saffron

This recipe pairs mango with cardamom, saffron and lemon zest. The pie shell is held together by the healthy Omega-3 and -6 oils in walnuts, and it's slightly salty and flavored with a hint of cardamom. This tart pie tastes best when served warm with a scoop of sweet vanilla soy ice cream on top. **1 (8-INCH) PIE (6–8 SERVINGS)**

Crust Ingredients

1¼ c. oats

1 c. chopped walnuts

2 Tbsp. honey

1 tsp. pure vanilla extract

1 tsp. freshly squeezed lemon juice

¼ tsp. salt

¼ tsp. ground cardamom

2 Tbsp. ice water

Filling Ingredients

¾ c. cold water

¼ c. cornstarch

4 c. sliced yellow mango (about 3 medium mangoes)

¼ c. honey (if you prefer a sweeter pie, use ½ c. honey instead)

1 tsp. grated lemon zest

1 Tbsp. freshly squeezed lemon juice

½ tsp. pure vanilla extract

½ tsp. ground cardamom

1 tsp. saffron, soaked in 2 Tbsp. organic unsweetened plain soy milk

¼ tsp. salt

Preheat oven to 350°F.

Make the crust: Place oats in a food processor and process until they turn into a fine powder. Next, add nuts, honey, vanilla, lemon juice, salt and cardamom, and process until the mixture forms a smooth paste. Pour in ice water and process just until mixture achieves a dough-like consistency. Do not overmix or crust will become too hard when baked. Remove mixture from food processor, scraping out remaining bits with a spatula. Using your hands, form into a dough ball, cover with plastic wrap, and place in the freezer for a half hour.

While you're waiting for the dough to freeze, make the filling: Combine cold water and cornstarch in a small bowl to make a slurry; stir together until smooth and also to break up any clumps. Set aside. Combine mangoes, honey, lemon zest, lemon juice, vanilla extract, cardamom, saffron mixture and salt in a large saucepan and cook on medium heat. Stir with a heatproof spatula, continuously folding mixture until honey has dissolved and the cornstarch slurry has adequately thickened the filling. The white color of the cornstarch slurry should completely disappear by the time the filling is finished cooking. Remove from heat and allow to cool.

Assemble the pie: Remove dough from freezer. If dough ball is too dry, add a small amount of water before rolling it out. For easy cleanup, spread waxed paper onto a clean, flat work surface. Using a rolling pin, roll out dough onto the waxed paper into a large circle formation until it's about a ¼" thick. Place an 8" pie plate face down onto the rolled-out dough, positioning it so that it's lined up properly with the dough. Lift up the waxed paper and gingerly flip it over so that the pie crust is now on top of the pie plate. Be sure to hold onto both the pie plate and the waxed paper while flipping them over. (If you don't feel comfortable doing this, you can also lift up the waxed paper and flip the dough over into the pie plate.) Mold pie crust to pie plate, pressing dough down to cover the bottom and sides of the plate. Perforate the sides and bottom of the crust with a fork so it won't rise up from the pie plate as it bakes. Place crust into the freezer again for 10 minutes. Then pre-bake the crust in the preheated oven for 15 minutes or until light golden brown. Keep checking on crust as it cooks to be sure it doesn't burn. Remove crust from oven and allow to cool for 10 minutes. Then pour in pie filling and bake in the oven at 350°F for 40 minutes. Allow to cool for another 10 minutes. Serve hot or warm, with a scoop of French vanilla soy or coconut milk ice cream on top.

Frosted Chocolate Fudge Brownies

Believe it or not, these brownies actually contain a wealth of healthy ingredients. They have zero refined sugar and are a lot lower in fat (and saturated fat content) than traditional brownies. The batter uses homemade oat flour (an excellent source of dietary fiber) and dates, which give the brownies their fudge-like consistency. The walnuts are a good source of omega-3s and -6s, while the almond butter in the frosting contains omega-6. Even better, these brownies actually taste like an honest-to-goodness traditional brownie but are much healthier for you. **9 LARGE (OR 16 SMALL) SQUARES**

Brownie Ingredients

1 c. oats

¼ tsp. salt

1 c. pitted medjool dates

5 Tbsp. raw unsweetened cocoa

2 tsp. baking soda

1½ c. organic, unsweetened plain soy milk

2 Tbsp. honey

1 tsp. pure vanilla extract

¾ c. chopped raw walnuts

¼ c. sliced almonds

Icing Ingredients

¼ c. light silken tofu

½ c. raw unsweetened cocoa

¼ c. raw almond butter

5 Tbsp. honey

2 Tbsp. unsweetened plain soy milk

⅛ tsp. salt

2 tsp. unbleached all-purpose flour

½ tsp. pure vanilla extract

sliced strawberries (to serve)

Preheat oven to 350°F.

Make the brownie batter: Process oats and salt in food processor for 1–2 minutes until finely ground into flour. (Take special care to grind the oats into a fine powder to ensure that the brownie batter is velvety smooth.) Add dates, cocoa powder and baking soda and process until well blended. (It's best to pulse in short bursts as you don't want the dates and other dry ingredients to clump together into a heavy mass.) Next, add soy milk, honey and vanilla and process until well blended and smooth. Turn off food processor. Fold in sliced almonds and chopped walnuts with a spatula until evenly distributed. Pour brownie batter into an 8" x 8" aluminum pan until evenly distributed. Bake in preheated 350°F oven for 20 minutes.

Make and spread the icing: While brownie is baking, mix together icing ingredients in a food processor until well blended, and refrigerate to allow icing to set. Allow brownie to cool completely. Remove icing from refrigerator and spread it over cooled brownie until evenly distributed.

Assemble and serve: Top with sliced strawberries. Allow brownie to set overnight in the fridge before serving. Cut into squares and serve.

Apricot-Papaya Pudding Parfait

This naturally sweet, low-fat parfait can be eaten as a dessert or as a post-exercise recovery snack. As a recovery option, it has the perfect combination of ingredients—plenty of antioxidants and electrolytes, a significant amount of carbs to replenish depleted glycogen stores, and protein to help repair muscle caused by exertion during exercise. So regardless of how you classify this recipe, how you decide to enjoy it is up to you! **4–6 SERVINGS**

Ingredients (MAKES 2 CUPS PUDDING)

1½ c. fresh apricots halves (about 4½ apricots)

¼ c. pitted medjool dates

½ c. diced papaya (if preferred, substitute with cantaloupe)

¼ c. unsweetened plain soy milk

pinch of salt

½ tsp. pure vanilla extract

1 tsp. ground cinnamon (or to taste)

¼ tsp. ground allspice

⅛ tsp. ground cardamom

Toppings

4–6 c. diced fresh apricots (about 1 c. per serving) (about 14–16 apricots)

2–3 c. vegan non-dairy whipped topping (or plain/vanilla soy yogurt) (about ½ c. per serving)

4–6 Tbsp. chopped walnuts (about 1 Tbsp. per serving)

⅛ tsp. ground cinnamon (for dusting)

Toss all of the pudding ingredients into a food processor and pulse until smooth. For one serving, add a layer of diced apricots to the bottom of a parfait or martini glass, followed by a layer of non-dairy whipped topping (or soy yogurt), and then a layer of pudding. Top parfait with more diced apricots and then sprinkle with walnuts and ground cinnamon. Repeat with remaining ingredients. Serve immediately.

THE GREAT VEGAN SWAP

So, you clipped a recipe you'd like to try out of a magazine or even downloaded it to your iPad and are all excited to make it for an upcoming dinner party, and then you realize it calls for eggs, milk, cheese, or even something more confusing to replace like buttermilk or gelatin. There's got to be an easy way to make some changes to the ingredients and make this a vegan meal, right?

Let's face it, most packages that have a recipe on the back don't offer a veg*n alternative for each of the ingredients, and unless you're getting recipes from veg*n sources, the chances of it containing ingredients that are outside of the scope of the vegetarian or vegan lifestyle are pretty high. That's where the Great Vegan Swap comes in—we'll take some of the most common ingredients found in most recipes or meals and give you some options to swap them out for veg*n-friendly alternatives!

Now, these swaps aren't necessarily a perfect 1-for-1 substitution, so they do require a little bit of finesse and practice to get the amounts just right. After all, we are talking apples and oranges a little bit!

Recipe calls for...	Swap for this!
Butter	Coconut oil, dairy-free non-hydrogenated margarine, vegetable shortening.
Buttermilk	Combine 1 c. of unsweetened soy milk with 1 Tbsp. of apple cider vinegar or freshly squeezed lemon juice. Stir well and let sit for about 10 minutes prior to using.
Cheese	From shredded cheese substitutes and dips to vegan cheese slices and crumbled feta, the market abounds with plenty of choices for an adequate cheese swap! Vegan feta cheese leads the charge, as the different consistencies allow it to be crumbled to closely resemble goat cheese or feta, cream cheese or even sliced pepper jack. Queso? Yes, we say so too!

Recipe calls for...	Swap for this!
Eggs, for baking	Applesauce, non-dairy yogurt, coconut milk, prunes and mashed bananas provide an adequate replacement in sweet treats. Non-dairy yogurt, coconut milk, and nut butters can be combined and whipped up with some puréed fruit or vegetables to create a consistency that's great for cakes and cookies. As listed in the other egg swaps, flax, egg replacer, tofu and starches are all useful ingredients.
Eggs, for cooking	Puréed tofu, potato starch, arrowroot and mashed white or sweet potatoes work well as do puréed pumpkin and squash.
Eggs, hard boiled	Firm tofu.
Eggs, scrambled	Soft tofu, best scrambled with some fresh veggies.
Egg whites	Combine 1 Tbsp. finely ground flaxseed mixed with 2–3 Tbsp. warm water. Powdered egg replacers mixed with water can be used for baking. Puréed soft tofu can provide a similar egg-like texture.
Gelatin	Many kosher gelatins (like KoJel, Carmel's Unsweetened Gel and Lieber's Unflavored Jel) and vegetable-derived starches (like cornstarch; potato, rice, tapioca, and cassava starches; arrowroot; and kudzu, also called Japanese arrowroot) are good vegan alternatives to traditional gelatin. Flaxseed, guar gum, fruit pectin and even chia seeds can also be used. In order for these ingredients to gel, they must be combined with water in the proper ratio. For example, use 2 Tbsp. arrowroot per 1 c. cold liquid; 1 Tbsp. flaxseed per 3 Tbsp. hot water; 1 Tbsp. cornstarch per 2 Tbsp. hot water. Be aware that some gelatin substitutes, like arrowroot, don't react well to heat, while others, like cornstarch, rice starch and tapioca starch do. Some, like fruit pectin, react well with either. Some substitutes, like guar gum, thicken quickly, so they should be added to dry ingredients first and then added to the wet. Others, like arrowroot, work better with acidic ingredients.

Recipe calls for...	Swap for this!
Heavy cream	Unsweetened coconut milk, coconut cream and vegan non-dairy creamers like soy or nut milk creamers.
Ice cream	Plenty of tasty alternatives are available in grocery stores. Soy, rice and coconut ice cream substitutes, or even fruit sorbet.
Meat, Poultry & Fish	Of course this is the biggest category to swap out for veg*n sources, and because of this there is a large cottage industry creating prepackaged menu items that will fit the bill. From mock burgers to imitation crab (often referred to as "krab"), there are so many different choices at the store to choose from. One word of caution, check the ingredients and calories, as imitations can often be hiding some ingredients or extra calories that you can do without.

Some excellent and extremely healthy do-it-yourself options are also very easy, like grilling up a portobello mushroom or swapping ground beef or turkey or legumes, tempeh, tofu or a textured vegetable protein (TVP).

Black bean or veggie patties are available in many different varieties and are becoming increasingly popular at burger joints, so you can maintain a compassionate lifestyle while on the go! |
Milk	There are plenty of options for this, although the consistency varies for each! Try soy milk, almond milk, hemp milk, rice milk and coconut milk.
Sour cream	There are a few store-bought tofu-based options on the market. Or make your own by blending 12 oz. firm tofu with 2 Tbsp. extra virgin olive oil, 2 Tbsp. lemon juice and a pinch of sea salt as needed.
Sugar	There is a plethora of artificial sweeteners on the market that can fit the bill, but there are more natural options that you can easily use too: evaporated cane juice, agave nectar, brown rice syrup, pure maple syrup, fruit syrup, fruit purees like banana, applesauce and blackstrap molasses.
Yogurt	Again, there are some tasty options available for purchase; coconut, rice, and soy yogurts are the most common and are offered in a wide variety of flavors.

VEGAN RESOURCES— JUST A CLICK AWAY

Living the vegan lifestyle, a compassionate, happy, healthy, balanced life in harmony with nature, can actually be improved with a little bit of technology. Whether it's new information, articles and updates, products created specifically for vegans or even insight to help you share your lifestyle choices with others in a deep and meaningful way, there are plenty of online resources to help guide you. You can find everything from a general overview to specifics of the lifestyle including nutrition, common foods, alternatives to eggs and dairy, vegan books and periodicals along with blogs, interviews, research and even a primer or two to help educate and prepare you for debates with well-intentioned (or some not so well-meaning) meat-eaters who question your choices and the vegan lifestyle in general. Of course, you're not necessarily trying to prove your life choices to anyone, but it never hurts to have a well-reasoned response.

*Helpful Links—General Veg*n Information*

The Vegetarian Resource Group
www.vrg.org
The registered dietitians and physicians at the Vegetarian Resource Group provide a great deal of information and support for the veg*n community through their website. From nutritional facts to recipes for adults and children, it is an extremely useful resource for families embracing the veg*n lifestyle together.

An outstanding example of the VRG's usefulness can be found in the "Vegan in a Nutshell" page that's also available as a downloadable PDF. Both the site and the handout provide answers about veganism at a glance while also offering in-depth knowledge to help educate others about the nutritional choices that vegans abide by.

Vegan.com
Packed with tons of resources for maintaining a vegan lifestyle, Vegan.com can help you find everything from what to make for dinner or where to dine out to the best vegan-friendly clothing brands and styles. This site is a great place to start for those who are new to veganism or are just curious about it. Their tagline, "Cutting through the BS," sets the tone immediately when you visit the site; the vegan resources are straightforward and simple to find.

Vegan.com offers several inexpensive books, including the digital version of *The Ultimate Vegan Guide* by Erik Marcus for less than a dollar; the first edition is free online at www.vegan.com/ultimate-vegan-guide.

Ethical Planet
www.EthicalPlanet.com

Ethical Planet is a friendly resource for individuals who are "vegan curious" as well as for vegan enthusiasts to get trustworthy information on how to lead a healthy and happy vegan lifestyle.

Ethical Planet's "The Upsides and Downsides of Being a Vegan" provides a simple, quick overview of some pros and cons of adopting the vegan lifestyle, and they recommend anyone who's not sure about making this important decision check it out first.

PETA, People for the Ethical Treatment of Animals
www.PETA.org

The high-profile PETA, with dozens of celebrity spokespeople and activists championing the cause of stopping animal cruelty, does not shy away from the spotlight when they have the opportunity to bring about change. Their mission statement, "Animals are not ours to eat, wear, experiment on, use for entertainment or abuse in any way," sums up their position. They provide a multitude of resources, information and research on living a compassionate, healthy lifestyle while respecting animals.

PETA's Vegetarian/Vegan Starter Kit includes the quiz entitled "Meet Your Meat," along with free vegan recipes, a 30-day pledge to be vegan and interactive resources you can share with your friends.

VegSource
www.VegSource.com

This site encompasses many great topics about the vegetarian and vegan lifestyle, including blogs, videos, health and lifestyle information. There's even a celebrity section that always has some interesting articles about vegans in Hollywood. The site also details what they are doing to better the world around them through education. This site is a one-stop shop for a wealth of veg*n information, articles, research and community feedback.

Happy Cow
www.HappyCow.net

Happy Cow is an amazing searchable database of vegan or vegan-friendly restaurants and stores worldwide. The site is especially helpful when you are traveling; it provides accurate vegan dining information no matter where you're visiting. It is highly recommended if you travel or eat out often.

VegNews.com

A very attractive magazine-format website, *Veg News* is a big-time online publication that covers food, travel, what's happening in the vegetarian/vegan community, news and so much more. *Veg News* has a plethora of interesting articles, guides, votes, tips and even "veg jobs" to possibly make your lifestyle choice part of your full-time employment!

Vegan Essentials
VeganEssentials.com

Owned and operated by vegans, this online shop will help you find virtually any type of vegan product that you could ever need. With over 1200 vegan products in stock, they carry everything from make-up and clothing to vitamins and books—you name it, they have it!

Vegan Bodybuilding
VeganBodybuilding.com

Let's get real—when most people think of bodybuilding, veganism is usually not the first thought that enters their mind. Vegan Bodybuilding covers news, training tips, lifestyle primers and articles, and especially supplements and all of the nutritional needs of a vegan athlete and bodybuilder. This site is a fantastic source for vegan supplements, proteins and what ever else you could ever possibly need to enhance and develop your physique while maintaining a compassionate lifestyle.

Some Good Examples of Regional Vegan Websites

Are you new to an area or new to the vegan scene and need to find local events, grocers or restaurants? A general site like Happy Cow (listed above) can be fantastic for locating vegan-friendly establishments nationwide, but sites dedicated to specific cities or states provide even more up-to-date happenings and can be your source to find some real local gems.

West

It should come as no surprise that California has several incredibly informative and useful vegan-centric websites. After all, the West Coast is home to many veg*n hot spots. PETA has rated San Francisco as one of the top-three vegetarian-friendly cities in America for several years!

Simple and straightforward, **vegSF.com** focuses on vegetarian and vegan-friendly restaurants, groceries, services and organizations all around the Bay Area.

A veggie-friendly trip to the City of Angels is well-served by **VegParadise.com**, a non-profit vegan web magazine serving the LA area, complete with a calendar of local vegan lifestyle happenings, restaurants, food markets, cooking classes, farmer's markets and more!

If you happen to be in SoCal and are in the mood for fresh and delicious veg*an fare delivered to your door, **VeginOut.com** should be your first click. They provide a weekly menu of entrees, soups, side dishes and even desserts that can be delivered fresh!

Northwest

Two of the top-three vegetarian-friendly cities in the U.S. are in the Pacific Northwest: Portland, Oregon, and Seattle, Washington. Based out of Seattle, the following are just two examples of regional sites that provide great features on local people, places and events for individuals who are living the vegan lifestyle. As a Seattleite, these sites are near and dear to Ben's heart. On **SeattleVegan.com**, you'll find an extremely helpful vegan grocery section that allows you to search aisle-by-aisle in some local grocery stores through a list of nearly every vegan grocery item that they stock! If you're looking more than just vegan food (although they provide resources for that as well!), **VeganScore.com** also is a one-stop site to learn more about Seattle vegan fashion, people and parties. This is truly a community-oriented online source for the Seattle vegan lifestyle.

Southwest

Based in Tucson, Arizona, **VeganOutreach.org** is a nonprofit organization working to end cruelty to animals and provide resources such as handouts and illustrated booklets that have been translated into dozens of different languages and distributed all over the world. Their outreach programs include "Adopt a College," which helps further educate students about compassionate living at colleges and universities across America.

Midwest

The Windy City has quite a few veggie-friendly websites and community resources. Two Meetup .com groups, VeganChicago.com and ChicagoVeg.org, are community-based sites where veg*ans can find happenings with local like-minded people. **VeganChicago.com** has existed for over a decade and boasts thousands of members in the area. It's a vegan support network that provides connections, resources and "unadulterated pure vegan awesomeness" for Chicagoans. **ChicagoVeg.org** helps to organize fun and educational events for vegans and non-vegans alike where all are welcome to express their opinions and socialize in a non-judgmental community.

East Coast

Living in or traveling through the Big Apple? By their own admission, **SuperVegan.com** is a "shockingly ambitious website made by vegans for vegans" and features the "Amazing Instant New York City Vegan Restaurant Finder" front and center on their website, and with just one click, nearly 100 results are instantly plotted on a map of Manhattan with the address, phone number, reviews and even a color-coded system for you to immediately tell how vegan the establishment is based on their marker on the map.

South

Listing nearly all of the restaurants in south Florida divvied up by county, **VegSouthFlorida.com** is a no-nonsense site for veg*ns to find healthy, delicious and animal-free meals from Key West to Palm Beach and all the cities in between. Each recipe has a write-up based on the amount of veg*n-friendly menu items, fare type and quality, as well as atmosphere.

The Vegetarian Society of Georgia, **VegSocietyofGA.org** focuses on healthy and humane living, and features links to other helpful sites and even an online video archive with nutritional information and cooking demonstrations. Member discounts at local veg*n-friendly restaurants and businesses, community events and even a printable leave-behind card to encourage your local restaurants to offer more vegetarian and vegan fare are just a few of the resources you can find on this helpful, friendly community site.

In Texas, **VeganAustin.org** is proud to state that "Vegans Rock Austin." The community is built around veg*n social interaction, and they list a calendar of many events and feature forums for the sharing of tips, recipes and the hottest new spots, as well as reviews, ratings and even uploads of photos from the restaurants so uses can find "the best vegan grub in town."

Recommended Books and Articles

To say this is an extremely small sampling of some of the amazing articles or publications on the vegan lifestyle is an obvious understatement, so consider these few examples as a mere primer and then explore some of the great resources you'll find in the more "general" websites above.

How to Win an Argument with a Meat-Eater
www.vegsource.com/news/2009/09/how-to-win-an-argument-with-a-meat-eater.html
We'd prefer if this article were titled "How to Educate Meat-Eaters about the Vegan Lifestyle," but it does get right to the point. The article focuses on helping to empower vegans when speaking with others who don't understand or accept your lifestyle and belittle it. Talking with carnivores about a plant-based diet is not always a simple conversation to have; studying the points in this article just might make it a little easier.

Harvard University's Vegan Dining Guide
www.dining.harvard.edu/vegvgn
While many of us (including the authors) may not have studied at prestigious Ivy League universities like Harvard, we can surely benefit from the information they provide on their website.

Compassionate Cook
CompassionateCook.com
Colleen Patrick-Goudreau, the author of multiple well-received vegan cookbooks and host of a very popular vegan podcast *Food for Thought*, runs this website. It offers information on everything vegan, from talking to strangers about veganism to how to make the best vegan meal possible. This is a great resource for those interested in sampling the vegan lifestyle, newly minted vegans and veteran vegans.

Finding Ultra, **by Rich Roll**
www.richroll.com/finding-ultra

"Rejecting Middle Age, Becoming One of the World's Fittest Men and Discovering Myself" is the subtitle and a great summation for Rich Roll's book that illustrates the amazing transformation of an overweight 40-year-old to an endurance athlete capable of completing some of the most elite and daunting tasks on the planet. Not content with merely finishing one Ironman-distance triathlon, Roll pushed the limit to five times that distance and more. An incredible true story and a must-read.

Eat & Run, **by Scott Jurek**
www.ScottJurek.com

Extremely well-known in endurance running as the greatest ultrarunner in the world, Jurek's accomplishments are that of legend: Winning the Western States Endurance Run, a 100-mile race through unbelievably rugged terrain with tens of thousands of feet of elevation change—while setting a course record along the way. He has set a new American record of running the equivalent of 6.5 marathons in 24 hours, over 165 miles! Jurek shares his upbringing in a meat-eating family and his conversion to veganism and his iron will and mentality of thinking of food as our fuel. Jurek is a truly exceptional athlete and human being, and *Eat & Run* should be on any athlete's must-read list.

CONVERSIONS

Measure	Equivalent	Metric
1 teaspoon	n/a	5.0 milliliters
1 tablespoon	3 teaspoons	14.8 milliliters
1 cup	16 tablespoons	236.8 milliliters
1 pint	2 cups	473.6 milliliters
1 quart	4 cups	947.2 milliliters
1 liter	4 cups + 3½ tablespoons	1000 milliliters
1 ounce (dry)	2 tablespoons	28.35 grams
1 fluid ounce	2 tablespoons	30 milliliters
1 pound	16 ounces	453.49 grams
2.21 pounds	35.3 ounces	1 kilogram
325°F/350°F/375°F	n/a	165°C/177°C/190°C

INDEX